Date: 2/2/22

DOES IT HURT
WHEN I DO THIS?

DOES IT HURT WHEN I DO THIS?

An Irreverent Guide to Understanding Injury Prevention and Rehabilitation

MARK SALAMON

ROWMAN & LITTLEFIELD
Lanham • Boulder • New York • London

Published by Rowman & Littlefield
An imprint of The Rowman & Littlefield Publishing Group, Inc.
4501 Forbes Boulevard, Suite 200, Lanham, Maryland 20706
www.rowman.com

6 Tinworth Street, London SE11 5AL, United Kingdom

British Library Cataloguing in Publication Information Available

Library of Congress Cataloging-in-Publication Data
Names: Salamon, Mark, 1964- author.
Title: Does it hurt when I do this? : an irreverent guide to understanding injury prevention and rehabilitation / Mark Salamon.
Description: Lanham : Rowman & Littlefield Publishing Group, 2021. | Includes bibliographical references and index. | Summary: "Mark Salamon integrates current scientific literature with his own twenty-five years of experience as a physical therapist to produce this humorous "owners manual" for the human body. Far from a dry guide, this entertaining read teaches readers how to maintain and restore good health, and can be referenced again and again when injuries arise"— Provided by publisher.
Identifiers: LCCN 2020048565 (print) | LCCN 2020048566 (ebook) | ISBN 9781538149027 (cloth) | ISBN 9781538149034 (epub)
Subjects: LCSH: Wounds and injuries—Treatment. | Wounds and injuries—Prevention.
Classification: LCC RD131 .S25 2021 (print) | LCC RD131 (ebook) | DDC 617.1—dc23
LC record available at https://lccn.loc.gov/2020048565
LC ebook record available at https://lccn.loc.gov/2020048566

For my brother,
who had to take his leave too soon

CONTENTS

Part IV: Treatments for Injuries

INTRODUCTION

On a winter morning in 2010, a fifty-five-year-old former college football player named Frank Ward showed up on my schedule for a physical therapy evaluation. He had not yet agreed to use a cane, and he walked with a pronounced limp as he struggled to move his 6-foot-4, 270-pound frame across the clinic to the exam room. He told me the story of how he developed a condition called peripheral neuropathy as the result of an adverse reaction to a medication. He had been an elite athlete in his youth and had continued to work out at a high intensity level until very recently. He loved to run, cycle, lift weights. These activities fueled him, made him feel alive. Now he could not walk up a flight of stairs without help, and one of his many doctors told him that he would likely end up in a wheelchair.

I will talk more about Frank's story later, but for now I will give up the ending: Frank did not end up in a wheelchair. In fact, he now competes in three-mile road races. I was Frank's physical therapist for the better part of two years, and I wish I could boast that I was single-handedly responsible for his success, but I cannot. Frank had the force of personality to conquer the grueling test of endurance known as the American healthcare system. He worked with his treating clinicians—and willed them to work with him—as a team. He asked a thousand questions. He took control of his situation. He did the things that separate those who achieve great outcomes from those who suffer poor outcomes.

A patient like Frank comes around once or twice in a physical therapist's career, but his lessons apply to everyone, not just those with devastating medical conditions. You and I are more likely to sustain injuries that are not nearly as overwhelming. I spend most of my days helping the competitive weight lifter who strained his back attempting to pick up a paper clip, the retired NASA engineer who injured his knee chasing his self-propelled lawn mower across his backyard, or the young mother who accidentally used olive oil to make homemade bath oil and got so slippery that she fell on her shoulder trying to get out of the bathtub. These are the everyday people who summon the courage and fortitude needed to publicly admit how they were injured and enter a system where the treatment you receive depends largely on what type of doctor you happen to see. A family doctor will give you drugs, a surgeon will cut you open, a chiropractor will crack your back, a physiatrist will stab you with needles, and a naturopath will try to sell you $1 trillion worth of supplements. With so many options to choose from, it is not always easy to decide which treatment sounds the least damaging.

Most people start with their primary care physician, or family doctor. Primary care physicians are trained to refer you to the specialist that will maximize the number of subsequent specialists you will need to see. If you bypass this step and stumble around on your own, you may accidentally land on the right specialist on the first try and deprive yourself of several of the above character-building experiences.

Even if you make this novice mistake, our system has backup measures that prevent your out-of-pocket costs from falling dangerously low. These protocols ensure that even if you only go to one doctor, you will be subjected to a battery of tests such as X-rays, MRIs, CAT scans, ultrasounds, urine analyses, blood tests, and palm readings. These miracles of modern technology can detect just about anything abnormal, so chances are the results will come back and your doctor will say something like, "Everything looks normal, so I have no idea why it hurts."

When this happens, there is a good chance that your doctor will send you to physical therapy, because that's where many doctors send patients when they have no idea what to do with them. That is where I come in. As a trained physical therapist, I use gentle modalities to reduce tension and relieve pain. A typical session might involve a soothing hot pack, a relaxing massage, deep-breathing techniques, cocktails, and a bedtime story. At least that is what I tell patients in order to convince them to come to their first appointment. Then, when they are at my mercy on the exam table, I confront them with the grim reality that the real world of physical therapy involves me grabbing their extremities and bending them into positions they have not been in since their trip down the birth canal. Patients are often surprised to learn that these maneuvers have actually been shown to reduce pain and relieve tension. After I administer this type of discomfort all day, I come home totally relaxed with absolutely no urge to argue with my wife or yell at my kids. I feel blessed to live in a country where it is legal to obtain a license and earn a salary to torture people. These patients typically thank me with a level of enthusiasm that is in direct proportion to the amount of pain that I inflict. They often bring me home-cooked meals or gift certificates to expensive restaurants. One patient tried to give me a bike. So as you can see, one of the best ways to relieve stress and lead a healthy life is to become a physical therapist. At times, physical therapy also benefits the patients as well.

An additional bonus is that physical therapy, unlike pharmaceuticals, doesn't cause dry mouth, constipation, dizziness, weight gain, nausea, hives, bulging eyeballs, oily discharge, memory loss, or erections lasting more than four hours. The downside, however, is that physical therapy can be expensive. If you don't have insurance coverage, the cost is usually about $75 per visit. If you are lucky enough to have coverage, your out-of-pocket cost might run you only $75 per visit. But at a fraction of that price, you can buy this book and learn how to perform most of your physical therapy at home. Think of it as an Ikea instruction manual that teaches you to put together a piece of furniture every bit as elegant as a handmade piece. You don't have to be MacGyver. Anyone can do this. In today's healthcare environment you have to be your own advocate, and often you have to also be your own doctor, nurse, pharmacist, nutritionist, and yes, physical therapist. It took me three years of graduate school to learn how to be a physical therapist, but quite honestly most of that time was spent learning how to impress people at parties by saying words like "dysdiadochokinesia." You really don't need to know how to do this in order to inflict basic physical therapy on yourself, so you should be able to learn the fundamentals in just a few weeks.

WHY I WROTE THIS BOOK

Several years ago, I was treating a patient for a low back injury. He was lying facedown on the treatment table while I ground my knuckles into the muscles surrounding his spine. This treatment melted away his tension and caused him to utter a variety of expletives at a gradually increasing decibel level. When other patients started to sneak out the back door, this was my usual sign that the therapy had reached its maximal benefit, so I decided to conclude the treatment. The patient then sat up and said to me, in all seriousness, that he was afraid to have the back surgery that he needed because his cousin had back surgery and the surgeon accidentally touched the wrong nerve in his back and his eyeball popped out.

This is an example of what I have to listen to all day. So during a typical shift, I might get five or six minutes when I don't have to explain things like why you don't have to worry about your eyeball popping out, or your heart shaking loose, or your nose hair bursting into flames. I use this time wisely so that I don't fall behind on the most important part of patient care: electronic record keeping. If you have been to a doctor recently, you know all about this. A typical doctor visit starts with a fun-filled hour at the front desk where you fill out forms similar to those needed for a mortgage, only longer. You spend the next hour in the waiting room reading every issue of *People* magazine dating back to the Renaissance. A medical assistant with a laptop then escorts you to the treatment room and immediately starts typing your entire medical history starting with your first bowel movement. This is the same history you filled out at the front desk, but the highly trained assistant knows that there is no way you will remember having done something that long ago.

The medical assistant then hands you a gown and leaves you alone to undress and figure out how to tie the gown. There is no instruction because the medical assistant has no idea how to tie the gown. Heart surgeons have no idea how to tie the gown. Is this the front? The back? The top? The choice of which private part of your body to leave exposed to the world is entirely up to you.

At some point, usually after about forty-five minutes, a physician assistant barges into the room, glances at the tangled mess you are wearing, asks you why you came, and types with blistering speed on the same laptop the story of your life that would rival in length the entire Harry Potter series. When this is complete, the physician assistant assures you that the actual physician will be with you momentarily.

Sometime during this wait the night cleaning crew comes in and dusts the cobwebs off your stiffening body and freshens you up before the cheerful doctor comes in and asks, "So, what brings you here today?" While you talk, the doctor resumes the competitive speed-typing started by the assistant. When this is complete, the doctor sends you on your way because your injury has long since healed on its own.

If you are lucky enough to still have an injury after your doctor visit, you may be referred to me for physical therapy. If this happens, I will start your first session with a detailed evaluation. I will ask you to describe exactly what happened. I will ask you about your medical history and all medications. I will ask you what you do for a living, what you do for fun, and how your injury affects these activities. I will examine your injured body part. I will measure your strength and range of motion. I will analyze the way you walk. I will instruct you in exercises and perform hands-on stretching techniques. And after all this, when you come back for your second visit, even if it is the very next day, there is a good chance that I will look at you and not remember anything about your injury.

Some people call this "having a senior moment," but this type of thing has been happening to me since I was five, and I'm a little tired of all these "seniors" getting all the special treatment. So I propose that we change the official terminology to "idiot moment" to be more inclusive of people like me.

At this point, you may be asking yourself, "Why did I buy a book written by such a moron?" Trust me, you will probably have this thought more than once. And when you do, I want you to remember my earlier words of wisdom: This book is way cheaper than your copay.

But the point is, it's not the doctor's fault that your appointments take six hours, and it's not my fault that I can't remember anything about your injury. It's the insurance company's fault! They force all of this electronic documentation upon us, and it takes up 90 percent of our time and brain space. I too have this computer that I wheel around with me, and I have to use every spare second to type in every detail of every patient visit. It is impossible to keep up without world-class typing skills and, more importantly, macros. Macros are to record keeping what nail guns are to house building. If I program enough macros into my computer, I can type eight thousand words per minute. The trick is to get these macros to make sense when they are all strung together, so the note looks like it was written by an actual human being. I see chart notes that look like this:

> She states the pain is moderate. She is currently experiencing. Physical therapy referral evaluation and treatment. Right foot. Hold for—scheduling requested for. Follow up visit in. ICE. Comfortable shoe. Patient referred for. STOP physical therapy. Patient to continue physical therapy.

Notes like these give lawyers erections that last way more than four hours.

The other problem with macros is that I may type a perfectly normal sentence, and part of a word just happens to be a macro that someone in another office programmed into the system. So I type, "Patient did well with gait training today with hemi-walker," and what appears in the note is, "Patient did well with gait training today with I applied cortisone cream manually to relieve hemorrhoidal itching-walker."

But back to the reason why I wrote this book. Like the man who was afraid his eyeball would pop out, many of my patients do not understand their injuries or why they were sent to physical therapy. Doctors and therapists strive to look up from their computers long enough to explain injuries using appropriate amounts of detail, and this is difficult. All patients are unique, and they understand different levels of detail. Some patients ask a lot of questions, others don't ask any questions, and many believe they understand when they really do not.

Some patients have already seen several doctors or therapists and report that each gave a different explanation. And then there's the internet, which can further compound the confusion.

Clinicians have a responsibility to properly educate all patients. We don't always get it right, myself included. This is a problem. We should get it right every time. My experiences and mistakes over the last twenty-five years have taught me that when I use simplistic explanations, like "Your back is really screwed up," I get it wrong. When I use technical explanations and medical jargon in an effort to appear more intelligent than I actually am, I get it wrong. But when I focus on the basics, I get it right.

When I focus on the basics, I respect the patient's intelligence and ability to understand. When I focus on the basics, I explain in plain language the anatomy, how each part functions, how the parts function together, how the injury disrupts this system, and how physical therapy helps. When I focus on the basics, I hear the following sentence with incredible regularity: "That makes total sense; why didn't anyone explain that to me before?"

So this book is about the basics. You cannot fully understand what you hear from a healthcare professional, what you read in the news, or what you see on the internet without a solid understanding of the basics.

Frank never gave up until he understood the basics. He inspired me to never give up until every one of my patients understood the basics. He inspired me to write.

I will teach you how your body works. I will teach you how injuries affect your body and how your body responds. I will teach you how your body heals and how physical therapy improves healing. And I will teach you the fundamentals of rehabilitation.

I know that some therapists will argue that it is irresponsible to suggest that people follow physical therapy instructions from a book. They will say that there is no substitute for hands-on evaluation and treatment by a skilled, licensed therapist who can pick up details of each person's unique biomechanical structure and movement in order to prescribe the correct treatment. I wholeheartedly agree, and I have two things to say in my defense. First, this book is meant to enhance the patient-therapist relationship, not replace it. I would consider it a blessing if every one of my patients came to me having read a book like this. Second, and I know every therapist out there has seen this, doctors sometimes choose not to send patients to therapy, instead handing them a sheet of paper with exercises on it and saying, "Go home and do these." No instruction. No supervision. No understanding of why or how the exercises work. If that happened to my mother, I would want her to have, at the very least, a basic understanding of the fundamentals that this book provides.

If you sustain an injury, do not use this book to treat yourself before you see your doctor to determine the exact nature of your injury and what restrictions you should follow. This is a very important step that is necessary to avoid potentially dangerous medical complications, such as you suing me. I previously mentioned the time needed to actually see your doctor. To expedite this process, I recommend calling to set up the appointment a couple of weeks before you get injured.

WHY SHOULD YOU LISTEN TO ME?

Over the years, I have found that one of the best places to find peace and quiet and get things done is the men's room. This was actually more true in the old days. Back then, a public restroom was a simple place where the most advanced technology was the indoor plumbing. It wasn't a place for lazy people. I had to push a lever attached to the toilet to flush, turn a faucet to run the water, and actually crank this little handle to dispense paper towels. Today, the restroom is a living, breathing work of modern technology that does everything but send me alerts telling me when I have to go. The joy of clanking around with my papers and duffle bag has been replaced by neurotic fear that any wrong move will cause these modern sensors to trigger a toilet-flushing, water-running, soap-squirting, towel-dispensing, wind-blowing flurry of paranormal activity. Men throughout America now tiptoe around restrooms like neurotic burglars, and I am no exception. By the time I make it out of a modern men's room, I'm a nervous wreck. I once changed my shirt in a stall. The toilet flushed eight times. And not just residential-grade flushes. I'm pretty sure I could have flushed a bowling ball down that toilet.

So I sat in the restroom stall at the clinic one day, trying not to make any sudden movements, and a doctor walked in and called out, "Mark, are you in there?" Apparently, someone told him I was in there. I had to answer, just in case he recognized my shoes. He said, "I just wanted to talk to you about a patient when you get out." I asked him the patient's name so I could get my thoughts together, and he told me, and I asked something else, and he asked me something, and before I knew it, we were having a full-blown conference as I sat there on the toilet.

After this conference I felt two things: stunned and awkward. Stunned because this doctor managed to get out of there without setting off the paper towel dispenser, and awkward because, well, it was just a little weird. But the point is, I have learned that if I pay attention, I can learn something *anywhere*. I earned a bachelor's degree in mechanical engineering and a master's degree in physical therapy, passed the state board exam, and kept up with the latest research. But for twenty-five years I have also treated thousands of patients, listened to their stories, talked with doctors in men's rooms, watched them perform surgeries (not in men's rooms), sat with radiologists while they interpreted MRIs and X-rays, and treated my own injuries.

That's another advantage I enjoy as a physical therapist. When I sustain injuries, I can treat myself. No referrals, no copays. Nobody poking me and touching me. Some therapists like to treat each other's ailments, but I prefer self-treatments in the privacy of my own home. That is one of the reasons I didn't become, say, a proctologist.

I have learned a great deal from my own injuries. For example, several years ago I had a painful condition called plantar fasciitis, which I will discuss later in more detail, but for now let me just say that it felt like someone was sticking a knife into my heel. I had always instructed patients with plantar fasciitis not to run. So when I had plantar fasciitis, I decided, of course, to run—every day, for six months. It took me this long to confirm that running, in fact, was bad for plantar fasciitis. Just to be sure, I repeated this experiment a couple of years later and came to the same conclusion. (This book is way cheaper than your copay.)

In my defense, I am a healthcare professional, and healthcare professionals suffer from a compulsive urge to scientifically prove that everything they have ever learned was wrong. This is why it is so hard to keep up with what is healthy and what is unhealthy. News outlets report the results of the latest studies. A year later new studies show the exact opposite. A year after that they're back to the first ones. It is maddening, and it causes many people to become cynical. "Eat what I want, do what I want, and die when I'm supposed to" is a phrase I've heard from many patients who have reached their wits' end.

Accurate information is not readily available to the public. Critical analysis of research is not part of news reports, and the best and most important studies often don't make headlines. News outlets report studies that improve ratings, rarely scrutinizing methods, sample sizes, interpretation of results, or the funding sources' likely agendas. This tedious chore is left to healthcare professionals, who are responsible for relaying accurate information to their patients. I take this responsibility very seriously and tackle it with a large dose of common sense. Healthcare is scientific, but judgment and opinion still play a large part in every treatment decision. I have yet to meet two healthcare professionals who agree on everything, and it is often wise to seek a second opinion. This book contains my opinions. I am not always right, but I back up what I say with evidence, logic, and common sense.

WHY PHYSICAL THERAPY?

A book about physical therapy is more important now than ever because I am not qualified to write about anything else. But if that's not reason enough, consider the state of healthcare in America. Costs are soaring, yet more expensive treatments are not producing better results.[1] Many people do not have access to healthcare, and those who do often cannot afford the out-of-pocket costs. Employers struggle to provide insurance for employees and cover the costs for those who sustain injuries on the job. This system is not financially sustainable, so the future of healthcare must involve treatments that are less expensive and produce better outcomes. Research shows that physical therapy is one such treatment.

A 2015 study published in the *Annals of Internal Medicine* showed that patients who had physical therapy for spinal stenosis had outcomes equal to those who had surgery.[2] Another 2015 study in the journal *Health Services Research* showed that when physical therapy was the first line of treatment for low back pain, overall costs for the first year were 72 percent lower.[3] Data collected by the Bureau of Labor Statistics and MedRisk Industry Trends Reports from 2003 to 2017 documented that increased physical therapy utilization corresponded with decreased time away from work as a result of injuries.[4,5] Even the financial market industry published reports that supported physical therapy, including reports from Capstone Partners Investment Banking Advisors from 2016 and 2017 that stated that with "the ever-increasing burdens on an already troubled healthcare system, commercial carriers and government sponsored healthcare programs are switching to value-based reimbursements and efficacious cost-effective treatments such as physical therapy."[6]

Physical therapy is not like taking a pill. Patient and therapist must work together as a team and form a one-on-one partnership, because patients with more knowledge and understanding have much better outcomes. Patients who ask a lot of questions have much better outcomes. Patients who take control of their recovery have much better outcomes.

Injuries occur across all ages and demographics, so no matter who you are, there is a good chance that you or a loved one will need physical therapy. At some point in their lives, 90 percent of Americans experience low back pain.[7] One-third of school-age children who participate in sports sustain repeated injuries.[8] Fifty percent of recreational injuries result in medical treatment.[9] One-third of all people over age sixty-five fall each year.[10] Every day, thousands of people lose control of their lives as the result of injuries to themselves or their family members. Indeed, those who have to care for, transport, pick up supplies for, and arrange appointments for injured parents or children know that an injury to a family member can throw many lives into chaos.

At a time when you feel you have the least control, knowledge is an enormous asset in restoring your sense of control. If you understand your body, your injury, and how to improve your recovery, you will gain control. If you learn the basics of reasonable self-care at a point when economics is one of the biggest stresses in your life, you will gain control. If you learn how to keep your body healthy and decrease the chance of injury, you will gain control.

And if you manage to keep your sense of humor, you will gain control. You may notice a few wisecracks in these pages. I do this for your own good, because research shows that humor and laughter improve overall health and well-being.[11] So even though it is difficult, I recommend that you at least try to laugh at some of my jokes in order to take advantage of this important health benefit.

Injuries disrupt lives. Financial hardships exacerbated or even created by the American healthcare system disrupt lives even more. Many patients are frustrated. You may be frustrated. If I can relieve some of your frustration, lift your spirits with an occasional bad joke, and empower you with the knowledge you need to optimize health and speed up recovery, I will consider this book a success.

PART I

HOW A HEALTHY BODY WORKS

1

THE PARTS LIST

The human body is a machine, and the instruction manual for any machine starts with a parts list. As a mechanical engineer, I see the human body as a system of mechanical parts that can be compared to the parts of a man-made machine. These parts include frames (bones), cables (muscles and tendons), screws and other fasteners (ligaments), pulleys (joints), oil (synovial fluid), bushings (cartilage), shock absorbers (discs), and electric wires (nerves). However, as a physical therapist, I know that a living machine is much more complex than a man-made machine. A car, for instance, does not develop inflammation or scar tissue. An automated system does not feel emotions like anxiety or jealousy—the only known exception to this being my first GPS that intentionally, on several occasions, tried to kill my wife. (I finally had to break off the relationship. With the GPS, I mean.)

But even though the human body is vastly complex, its physical structure comprises mechanical parts, the "nuts and bolts," if you will. So I will start with a very brief description of these components. All of the details in the following chapters rest on this very basic, solid foundation.

NUTS AND BOLTS

Bones

Everyone knows what bones are.

Just kidding. Most people don't really know what bones are and think that they are simply made of hard, solid material. In fact, bones are dynamic, ever-changing tissues with blood flow, nerves, and a certain amount of flexibility. Bones are made up primarily of collagen, which is a structural protein. Different types of collagen combine to form the basic structures of virtually all connective tissues in the body, including tendons, ligaments, skin, hair, nails, and bones. Bones also contain calcium phosphate, which is a mineral that hardens this collagen framework and creates the solid structure of the skeleton.

Muscles

Muscles are also made up primarily of collagen, along with other structural proteins that are arranged in fibrous filaments that are twisted around each other in a complicated system that allows this tissue to contract and make itself shorter when stimulated by a nerve impulse. Using this ability to contract, muscles pull on bones to move or stabilize them. A muscle can only contract or relax. When a muscle contracts, it pulls. When a muscle relaxes, it stops pulling. A muscle cannot push.

Tendons

Tendons connect muscles to bones. Each end of a muscle tapers off into a tendon, which attaches to a bone. Tendons are also made up of different types of collagen. Tendons are tough and rubbery and can withstand high levels of tension. If you eat a chicken leg, the tendon is the part that triggers a gag reflex to hurl the contents of your mouth across the table.

Ligaments

Ligaments connect bones to bones. In the same way a set of hinges holds a door to a frame, a set of ligaments keeps the bones congruent and stable so that they move smoothly in the proper direction. The types of collagen in ligaments allow them to withstand even higher loads than tendons, which makes them very hard to stretch. If you bend chicken bones the wrong way, you will hear ligaments tearing. (You can learn a lot about the human body by eating chicken.)

Joints

A joint is the connection of two bones. A fibrous joint does not move because the bones are solidly fixed together, like the bones that form the skull. A synovial joint allows movement between the bones; it gets its name from synovial fluid, which is a clear liquid that bathes and lubricates the joint.

Joint Capsule

A joint capsule is a sheath that surrounds every synovial joint and functions to contain the synovial fluid, like a balloon full of water. It is made of the same collagen structure as a ligament. In fact, some ligaments blend into the joint capsule and combine to form one solid structure. There is no blood inside a joint, only synovial fluid. If a doctor uses a needle to drain fluid from a joint and there is blood in the fluid, this is a sign that there is a tear in a ligament or joint capsule that is allowing blood to leak into the joint.

Cartilage

Cartilage is the shiny white substance at the end of a bone where it makes contact with another bone. Cartilage is primarily made up of—you guessed it!—another combination of different types of collagen. Healthy cartilage is smooth and slippery to minimize friction between the bones as they move. A sudden traumatic injury or years of normal wear and tear over a lifetime can damage cartilage and create painful rough spots. The term "bone-on-bone" refers to a joint with nearly all of the cartilage worn away.

Bursa

A bursa is a thin sac of synovial fluid that lubricates and cushions the area between tendon and bone. A normal bursa sac looks like a sheet of cellophane. Excessive pressure on a bursa can be caused by things like prolonged kneeling or leaning on the elbows and can lead to inflammation called bursitis. An inflamed bursa can produce excessive synovial fluid and swell up like a balloon.

Meniscus

A meniscus is a pad of soft tissue that functions as a cushion between the bones of the knee joint. There are two in each knee, one on the inside (medial) and one on the outside (lateral). The meniscus protects the cartilage because its collagen composition makes it softer and more shock-absorbent than cartilage. A torn meniscus is often incorrectly referred to as a torn cartilage.

Labrum

A labrum is a cushion of soft tissue that lines the rim of the socket in a ball-and-socket joint, such as at the shoulder or hip. It is similar to the meniscus in the knee and softens the force of contact between the two bones.

Discs

Discs are shock absorbers located between adjacent spinal vertebrae. The outside of a disc is tough and rubbery. The inside is a gelatinous material made primarily of water and collagen that helps distribute the pressure evenly when the spine bends or twists.

Nerves

Nerves transmit electrochemical signals through the body. A single nerve contains thousands of microscopic "wires," or neurons. If a nerve is compared to a length of yarn, a neuron corresponds to an individual thread in the yarn. An actual neuron is much thinner than a thread of yarn, so thin that it is visible only through a microscope.

Each neuron performs one specific function. Some transmit signals that cause a muscle to contract. Some sense heat, others cold. Some sense light touch. Some sense dull pressure. Others sense burning, and so on. All of these individual neurons are clumped together in a single nerve, so pressure on one part of a nerve may cause shooting pain, while pressure on a slightly different part of the nerve may cause a tingling sensation. Microscopic differences in where each neuron is located can cause two people with identical injuries to have completely different symptoms.

HORMONES

The above "nuts and bolts" are important, but I will now describe more complex parts that are unique to organic, living machines, starting with hormones. Endocrine glands are organs that manufacture and secrete biochemical substances called hormones directly into the bloodstream, where they are carried quickly to the rest of the body. Hormones perform a wide variety of functions that are far more complex than those of mechanical devices. There are hormones for just about every occasion, so let's start with one of the most popular.

Testosterone

When our daughters were young, we went to an outdoor summer party. While the grown-ups stayed outside, the kids went down to the basement to play. After a while I decided it would be a good idea to check on them, so I went downstairs, and this is what I found: The boys were playing a game that consisted of them taking turns running at full speed across the room and slamming their bodies into the wall. The girls were standing there watching, with puzzled looks. Finally, one of my daughters asked, "Dad, what's wrong with them?"

This fun-loving behavior is the result of testosterone, which evolved millions of years ago because when humans lived in caves, males who exhibited this kind of behavior obviously increased their chances of survival. Testosterone is manufactured in the male testicles and, to a lesser extent, the female ovaries. Atmospheric conditions such as the presence of oxygen can stimulate a testosterone release in young males, and an opportunity to run at full speed into a wall can trigger a full-blown testosterone storm. Testosterone also improves survival rates of physical therapists by providing a steady supply of new patients with contact sports injuries.

Estrogen

I live with my wife, three daughters, a female cat, and a female dog, so I could write an entire book about estrogen. The female ovaries and, to a lesser extent, the male testicles produce and secrete estrogen, which is the female counterpart to testosterone. Estrogen improves verbal memory scores, widens the hips, and develops the breasts, while testosterone produces body hair, acne, and armpit odor. Sounds about right.

Human Growth Hormone

The pituitary gland, a small, pea-sized gland at the base of the brain, produces and secretes human growth hormone, or HGH, which makes humans grow. This is a distinct advantage in the animal kingdom. Unfortunately, it is also an advantage in the professional sports kingdom, which has led many athletes to illegally abuse synthetic versions of this hormone.

Endorphins

The pituitary gland also secretes more than twenty different types of hormones called endorphins in response to various stimuli. Endorphins are similar to opioids such as morphine. In fact, the term "endorphin" literally means "morphine-like." Endorphins inhibit pain signals in the brain and cause sensations of euphoria, so they are great hormones to utilize after a hard day of self-inflicted physical abuse caused by too much testosterone. Endurance athletes are very familiar with endorphins, as they create the famous "runner's high."

Adrenaline

Humans have two adrenal glands, one on top of each kidney. When the adrenal glands secrete adrenaline into the bloodstream, the arteries of the body constrict and the heart beats rapidly. This is the well-known fight-or-flight response, which has protected humans throughout history by preventing them from engaging in dangerous behaviors such as public speaking.

Cortisol

During stressful or dangerous situations, such as being near someone with too much testosterone, the adrenal glands also produce and release cortisol. Commonly known as the "stress hormone," cortisol shuts down digestion and increases heart rate, respiration rate, and blood pressure.

People under constant stress continually secrete cortisol into their bloodstreams, which can, over time, weaken their immune systems, stunt their growth, and cause hypertension, ulcers, depression, irritable bowel syndrome, insomnia, and compulsive disorders. Most Americans are already accustomed to these conditions because, according to modern television drug commercials, they are the same side effects that occur with virtually every medication on the market.

And There's More—Much More

There are approximately seventy-five different hormones that at any given moment could be circulating through the bloodstream at ever-changing concentrations and combinations. This makes treating a human body much more complicated than working on a machine made of only nuts and bolts. With a human, the nuts and bolts are important, but the mechanical logic is complicated by a continually changing mixture of chemical reactions created by hormones. This is not a human physiology textbook, but I included a list of all of these hormones and the organs that secrete them in appendix II. You do not need to know these off the top of your head, but my hope is that if you take a quick look at this list, you will get a feel for the enormous complexity of the human machine.

DEFENSE MECHANISMS

The human body is also equipped with mechanisms of protection that can confound the rehabilitation process. Hundreds of defense mechanisms protect the human body from outside threats. These systems include everything from immune cells that fight infections and diseases to pigments that protect the skin from harmful rays of the sun. Injuries can trigger three particular defense mechanisms that can sometimes spiral out of control and cause more problems than the injuries themselves. These mechanisms are muscle spasm, inflammation, and scar tissue.

Muscle Spasm

When the nervous system senses injury, it sends signals to the muscles that surround the injury to reflexively contract in order to brace and protect the area. This constant, involuntary contraction is called muscle spasm. This reflex is particularly robust with neck or back injuries and causes stiffness that makes movement uncomfortable.

Muscle spasm can also cause pain in the same way that a tightly clenched fist held all day long will make the hand very sore. A minor injury, or even a prolonged awkward position, can trigger muscle spasm that may produce more pain than the original injury itself. Muscle spasm can also persist and cause chronic pain long after the injury has healed.

Inflammation

Illness, disease, infection, allergic reaction, or injury can trigger inflammation, which is a series of biochemical reactions that initiate tissue repair. Most chemical reactions give off energy and heat, so inflammation can cause an injured body part to become hot, red, painful, or swollen. Acute or short-term inflammation is necessary and should start to subside in a few days as healing proceeds. However, chronic inflammation—which persists for weeks, months, or even years—can cause severe problems, including permanent tissue damage, chronic pain, and disability.

Scar Tissue

The body forms scar tissue during the cellular process of soft tissue repair. This scar tissue is necessary because it bonds the damaged tissue like glue. But for unknown reasons, the body sometimes produces too much scar tissue, which creates adhesions that bond structures that normally glide on each other. This scar tissue can also become hard and stiff, which makes it very difficult to restore normal range of motion. The body often produces excessive scar tissue after surgery. Chronic inflammation can also cause excessive scar tissue formation.

These protective mechanisms perform vital functions. But the problem is, they often go into overdrive and continue to work long after they should have stopped, like switches that get stuck in the "on" position. Later chapters will describe how to prevent these situations.

STRIVING FOR BALANCE

To review: the parts list includes nuts and bolts, hormones, and protective mechanisms. For these parts to work together efficiently, physical, mental, and emotional conditions must be balanced. Emotional trauma can affect hormone levels, which can trigger protective mechanisms, which can cause physical pain. Conversely, physical injury can cause pain, which can trigger protective mechanisms, which can alter hormone levels, which can create emotional distress. Every part connects to every other part, and treatments often fail because these connections between the mind and the body are overlooked. The next chapter will examine these relationships in more detail.

2

THE MIND-BODY CONNECTION

I made a startling discovery during my first year as a therapist, and my experiences over the ensuing twenty-five years have confirmed this finding: When I ask a patient to lie on their back, nine out of ten times they lie on their stomach. Similarly, when I ask them to bend their knee, they straighten it, and when I ask them to straighten their knee, they bend it. I used to get very frustrated at work. Several times a day I could be heard to say, "Bend your knee. No, bend. No, no, bend, bend. No, *bend your knee!*" (smack to the forehead). Then these patients would laugh and say, "Oh, you mean *bend.*"

It's not like I was asking them to stand on their head and sing "The Star-Spangled Banner." Just bend your freaking knee!

But these days I am much more relaxed, and when I want someone to bend their knee, I just ask them to straighten it.

This phenomenon illustrates the essence of the mind-body connection: The mind has a thought, and the body performs a random movement completely unrelated to that thought. I always thought that the mind-body connection would work much better if there were a direct relationship between the mind's thought and the body's action, and I believe that at some point in human history this relationship did exist. But the mind-body connection has eroded and atrophied due to several factors, one being technology.

High-tech machines now do most of the work that our brains used to do. Take smartphones, for example. Virtually every human being over the age of six months now carries around a tiny supercomputer with access to all of the information in the universe, so most of my patients can name every *American Idol* contestant dating back to the Bronze Age, but they can't remember what "bend your knee" means.

These machines have even taken over normal conversations, laughing at us as they playfully autocorrect our words to make our sentences wildly inappropriate. Before smartphones, the mind-body connection had to be fine-tuned. If the mind's thought was, "I am going to have a conversation," the body's actions often had to involve a number of simultaneous activities such as talking, walking, avoiding traffic, opening doors, negotiating escalators, and making direct eye contact. Today, if the mind's thought is, "I am going to have a conversation," the body's action is to squint into a tiny screen and walk directly into a glass door.

People driving their cars don't have to worry about directions anymore, thanks to an ingenious piece of modern technology called the GPS, or global positioning system. I do a lot of home visits, so I am a big fan of the GPS, which makes my life so easy that entire sections of my brain that used to be dedicated to reading maps and paying attention can be completely shut down or dedicated to more important tasks, like selecting a podcast. The downside is that my brain can no longer remember how to get anywhere—including the end of my driveway—so when my GPS crashes, I have absolutely no idea how to get home.

These situations do not bode well for our collective health. I do not propose that we do away with our smartphones and mobile devices, but we do need to pay more attention to our minds. We need to exercise our brains, which, like muscles, become stronger in response to work. When we perform crossword puzzles or brain teasers, learn new languages, or do things with our nondominant hands, we exercise our brains. And every time we talk instead of text, or drive without our GPS, we improve memory, build mind-body connections, and decrease our chances of walking into a wall or accidentally driving to Mexico.

In other words, brain exercises affect our bodies. But this connection goes the other way as well: Body exercises also affect our brains. In fact, some studies show that physical exercises improve brain function more than brain exercises do.[1] This explains why professional athletes are so much smarter than the general population. Okay, maybe that's a bad example. But the point is, it's all about circulation. Physical exercise increases heart rate, which forces more blood, nutrients, and oxygen into all of the body's tissues, including the brain.

Exercise has a profound effect on the two specific brain areas—the hippocampus and the prefrontal cortex—that are most susceptible to damage from degenerative diseases such as Alzheimer's. The hippocampus is a small structure deep in the brain that is involved in conversion of short-term memories to long-term memories. The prefrontal cortex is a large area in the front of the brain that performs executive functions such as planning, decision making, and problem solving. Exercise has been shown to actually *increase the size* of the hippocampus and prefrontal cortex, which improves brain function and protects against the devastating effects of degenerative diseases.[2,3]

So if the mind-body connection is healthy, the components of the machine—nuts and bolts, hormones, and defense mechanisms—will work together in a coordinated synergy. The next chapter will describe how to keep this machine working to its full potential.

PART II

KEEPING THE BODY HEALTHY

3

NUTRITION

As a physical therapist, I have dedicated my career to restoring health through strategic, specialized, and targeted exercise. Every day I prescribe exercise, correct exercise technique, adjust exercise programs as recovery proceeds, and convince patients that exercise is beneficial and if they just stick with it, they will one day not hate it quite so much. So it may surprise you to learn that in my opinion, the single most important thing you can do to maintain good health is not to exercise, but to eat the right foods and avoid the wrong foods.

I hear this line too many times: "I eat whatever I want because I work out so hard that I burn it off." This is nonsense. I have treated life-long exercise enthusiasts who look fit and healthy on the outside, while slow and steady damage is occurring on the inside by chronic conditions like high cholesterol, high blood pressure, type 2 diabetes, cardiovascular disease, and chronic low-grade inflammation. Not only do these conditions contribute to massive health problems in the long term, they also make injuries more likely to occur and more difficult to treat in the short term. Bodies fueled by processed foods that are high in calories, low in nutrients, and laden with chemicals exhibit poor circulation, decreased immune responses, and delayed healing, so they do not respond well to rehabilitation. I cannot in good conscience write an entire book about exercise and ignore nutrition. And I cannot write about nutrition without delving into the fascinating evolution of the standard American diet.

First, a disclaimer: I am not a trained nutritionist. The opinions I share are my own. They in no way represent the opinions of any corporate sponsors of this book, of which there are none. My opinions are informed by critical analysis of research, and I include references so you can check my sources.

So now that my butt is covered, let's start at the beginning of what I like to call the Golden Age of Diets: the 1950s. This was when one of the most trusted and ethical entities ever assembled—the federal government—unveiled the concept of the four food groups: meat, dairy, fruits/vegetables, and breads/cereals. Impartial scientists who just happened to be heavily influenced by the meat and dairy industries helped develop this paradigm[1] and succeeded in convincing Americans everywhere that half of everything they eat should consist of meat or dairy products.

Since breads and cereals made up only a quarter of this diet, the grain farming industry, understandably, felt slighted. So they spent years accumulating evidence that eating more grains and bread would result in better health, presented this to legislators in the form of monetary pressure, and in 1992 finally succeeded with the creation of the food pyramid.[2] This public health breakthrough recommended that Americans eat more than twice as much grain and bread than any other food group. This turned out to be a boon for business, especially businesses that sold weight-loss programs or diet books, which made millions of dollars by basically telling people to stop eating so much bread.

From 1992 to the present, these diets have been a major factor in the growth of the American economy, also known as pharmaceutical companies. Popular and beloved diets have included the South Beach Diet, which advocated eating before you got hungry so that the hunger didn't make you eat; the Paleo Diet, which simulated the diet that our caveman ancestors utilized to live to the ripe old age of twenty-five; and my personal favorite, the Atkins Diet, which basically said screw it, just eat all the eggs and bacon you want. (This diet's creator, Dr. Robert Atkins, personally demonstrated the efficacy of his diet by having a heart attack.)

America also achieved world leadership in creative diet names, including—and these are all real—the SparkDiet, Flat Belly Diet, Engine 2 Diet, Fertility Diet (only works in conjunction with having sex), and Supercharged Hormone Diet (works best in combination with Fertility Diet), to name just a few. These and other diets were wildly successful in creating what we now refer to as the obesity epidemic, as participants achieved levels of hunger that eventually compelled them to snack on things like Philadelphia tacos. (For those of you not from Philly, a Philadelphia taco is a cheesesteak wrapped in a pizza.)

The processed food manufacturing industry grew in parallel with the diet industry. To understand this evolution, we need to go back again to the 1950s, when food manufacturing companies set the health-conscious, altruistic goal of making huge amounts of money. But over time these companies changed their business models and established a new goal, which was to make much, much more than huge amounts of money. Several of these companies recently admitted that the secret to their success was the manipulation of salt, sugar, and chemical levels to cause cravings that effectively made their foods addictive.[3,4] This ingenious strategy enabled them to meet their obligations to their shareholders, who desperately needed this extra money to pay for their diabetes medications.

The only thing left to do was to pump beef cattle and dairy cows with anabolic steroids to speed up growth and milk production. This started with diethylstilbestrol (DES) in 1954, and by 2007 included estradiol, testosterone, progesterone, zeranol, trenbolone acetate, melengestrol acetate, and recombinant bovine growth hormone (rBGH).[5,6,7] With a food supply on a blood doping program that rivals that of the 1976 Russian weightlifting team, we now boast a patient population that is the envy of heart surgeons and cancer specialists throughout the world.

Recent years have seen a surge of research by scientists who have this crazy theory that the standard American diet may have something to do with our healthcare costs (double that of other industrialized countries) and our healthcare outcomes (worse than all of these countries).[8] These scientists propose that our healthcare costs would go down and outcomes would improve if Americans would only eat the right foods.

What are the right foods? Great question. The vast array of dietary options include:

Vegan—no animal products
Vegetarian—no meat
Carnivorous—only meat
Pescatarian—no meat except fish

Whole foods—real food in its natural form, no chemicals or pro-
cessing

Ketogenic—high fat, no carbs

Intermittent fasting—nothing

Fast mimicking—nothing, but actually something

Fruitarian—only fruit

Plant-based—mostly plant foods

Lactovegetarian—no meat or eggs; dairy okay

Ovo-vegetarian—no meat or dairy; eggs okay

Ovo-lacto-vegetarian—no meat; eggs and dairy okay

Semi-vegetarian—no meat except for once in a while

Kangatarian—no meat except for kangaroo meat

(I did not make that last one up.)

Pollotarian—no meat except for poultry

Fratatarian—no vegetables, fruit, nuts, beans, or whole grains; beer
and pizza okay

(Okay, I did make that last one up.)

Throughout the world, physicians, researchers, and scientists who dedicate their careers to the study of nutrition are at this very moment arguing over which of the above regimens represents the healthiest diet. Hundreds of studies support and refute nearly every possible viewpoint, so boiling the entirety of the research down into one conclusion is an arduous task. But nearly all of the researchers agree that all of the above diets (except the last one) are far superior to the standard American diet. Most researchers also agree, or at least concede, that no single diet is best for every person. Normal biochemical differences between people cause them to respond differently to different diets. The ideal diet for one person may cause significant health problems in another.

Having said this, a few major pieces of relatively new information are worth considering. This is certainly not exhaustive, but remember, this book is about basics.

RECENT RESEARCH

Meat

In 2015 the International Agency for Research on Cancer (IARC), which is the cancer agency of the World Health Organization, classified processed meat as a carcinogen and red meat as a probable carcinogen.[9]

A large body of research, including a 2019 study in the *European Heart Journal*, suggests that increased red meat consumption correlates with increased heart disease risk.[10]

Protein

The myth that meat is necessary for adequate protein intake has been proven wrong.[11] Many plant-based foods are packed with protein. The recommended daily allowance of protein is about 0.36 grams per pound of body weight, so consider the following example of a typical day in the life of a vegan. (Parentheses indicate grams of protein in each food.)

Breakfast: oatmeal (5g) mixed with chia seeds (5g), fruit (3g)
Snack: peanuts (10g)
Lunch: quinoa (8g) mixed with broccoli (5g) and corn (5g)
Snack: fruit (3g) mixed with sunflower seeds (10g)
Dinner: rice (5g) mixed with beans (15g), a potato (5g), and peas (8g)

This is not an enormous amount of food, but it contains 87 grams of protein, which is enough for a 240-pound man. Most Americans who eat meat consume almost double the recommended amount of daily protein, which can lead to long-term health risks.[12]

Dairy

The United States Department of Agriculture (USDA) recommends three servings of dairy products per day despite the fact that a preponderance of research correlates this much dairy consumption with high rates of several types of cancer, including prostate, breast, ovarian, and testicular.[13,14,15,16,17,18] Cancer rates increase with consumption levels as low as two servings per day, and continue to increase proportionally for those who consume three or more servings per day.

Increased dairy consumption correlates with increased risk of heart disease.[19,20]

Research refutes the popular belief that dairy products strengthen bones and ward off osteoporosis.[21,22,23] Countries with the highest dairy consumption have the highest osteoporosis rates.[24]

Sugar

Diabetes, obesity, cancer, and heart disease risks increase proportionally with processed sugar consumption rates.[25,26,27,28]

Processed sugar is absorbed directly from the stomach into the bloodstream. Most processed foods, even those labeled "healthy" by the manufacturers, contain processed sugar.

Fruit contains sugar, but the pulp of the fruit holds the sugar until it is well into the intestines, where it is metabolized and absorbed slowly without raising blood sugar levels. Some studies show no adverse effects in participants who eat fruit continually every day for several weeks.[29]

Supplements

Does the typical human body need quantities of nutrients that it can only get from pills or powders? No. Research shows that a proper diet provides sufficient quantities of nutrients.[30] Some people with dietary restrictions or medical conditions need to supplement, but otherwise, supplements are unnecessary and in many cases can be harmful.[31,32]

MY ADVICE

Based on current knowledge, it is clear that the best way to stay healthy and live a long life is to follow a strict vegan diet. *Wait—come back! I'm only kidding!* I would never insist that you do something so radical, mainly because there are many more great things in this book that I still want you to read. But I will give you my honest opinion: Based on current knowledge, I believe that for most people, the best way to stay healthy and decrease the chances for disease is to eat a plant-based whole foods diet.

Put simply, whole foods means real foods in their natural forms: no chemicals, additives, or supplements. Processed foods that come in plastic containers or as packets of powder are not whole foods. Apples, carrots, and peanuts are whole foods.

Plant-based means that most of what you eat should come from plants instead of animals. Plant-based foods are packed with nutrients that fuel your body, boost your immune system, and protect you against many diseases, including cancer and heart disease. Since different plant-based foods have different nutrients, the key to this type of diet is to eat a wide variety of foods. Don't count portions or calculate specific nutrient amounts in each food. If you eat mostly fruits, vegetables, nuts, beans, and whole grains (bread, rice, pasta, quinoa, corn, oats) you will get all the nutrients you need, and you can eat as much of these foods as you want.

A plant-based whole foods diet can include small amounts of animal products such as organic meats, eggs, and dairy products. Quantity is the key. The standard American diet contains gigantic amounts of animal products, and this quantity causes the above-mentioned health risks. Fish is healthier than chicken, and chicken is healthier than red meat. Many studies show that moderate amounts of fish have beneficial health effects, while processed meats such as hot dogs and pepperoni significantly increase risks of disease.

Plant-based foods provide the fuel on which most human bodies thrive, so many people who adopt plant-based whole foods diets gradually crave more plant foods and eventually transition to vegan diets. These do not work well for everyone. As I said before, every human body has different biochemistry. But many people report feeling their very best on vegan diets. If you have heart disease or a family history of heart disease, you may want to seriously consider veganism, as it is the only diet that has been shown to reverse arterial blockages that cause heart attacks.[33] One famous example is Bill Clinton, who credits this diet with saving his life. Understandably, many people with heart disease still see a vegan diet as extreme and may elect to proceed with the more conservative, less radical approach of having their rib cage torn open with a circular saw.

If you do decide to try a vegan diet, you must take a B12 supplement. This is one of the few dietary situations when supplements are necessary. As I mentioned previously, unnecessary supplements at high doses can cause harm, as the following story illustrates.

About ten years ago I was the typical American vitamin taker: I was never sure if they really helped, I just figured they couldn't hurt. Since taking one pill at a time would have put me way behind schedule, I would take a handful of seven or eight pills—some of them big enough to be used as bookends—and swallow them all at once. (This book is way cheaper than your copay.) Naturally, one got stuck sideways in my esophagus one morning, which earned me an ambulance ride to the hospital in my jammies. Luckily it wasn't in my windpipe, or you would be doing something much more productive than reading this book right now.

After this episode, I decided to stop taking vitamins because those things can kill you. I figured this would be a good way to test whether or not they were beneficial. After a couple of weeks, the first thing I noticed was that I did not have to go to the emergency room. The second thing I noticed was that I felt absolutely no different. Everything, including my workouts, sleep quality, and energy level all felt the same.

You should take large supplement doses only if there is a medical reason and in consultation with your doctor. Do your research. And please, don't try to swallow eight pills at once.

4

SLEEP

When my daughters were just babies, everyone would ask me, "Hey Mark, how are those little girls? Mark? Are you okay? Mark? Wake up, Mark! Mark! (violent shaking) *Does anyone know CPR?*"

My girls kept me awake for fourteen months straight. I shouldn't say that. I took a twenty-minute nap once a day at around three in the morning. That's pretty much all I remember, so I have experienced the effects of sleep deprivation firsthand. (I also took naps sitting at red lights. I don't recommend this.) It wasn't a particularly healthy lifestyle. Sleep deprivation can inhibit tissue repair and disrupt body chemistry, throwing the delicate balance of pain modulators out of equilibrium. So when it comes to injury rehabilitation, sleep is just as important as nutrition.

Fatal familial insomnia is an extreme condition that shows how essential sleep really is. This inherited disease causes the part of the brain that modulates sleep to slowly atrophy. It usually strikes in midlife and makes sleep physiologically impossible. It is a horrible death. Paranoia progresses to hallucinations and convulsions. Organ systems shut down, and within a few months the brain shuts down and death occurs. Sleep is absolutely essential for life. It is possible to tough it out temporarily, but prolonged sleep deprivation can cause severe organ damage or even death.

The frustration with sleep is that the more you worry about it, the harder it is to fall asleep, so I'm not sure why I decided to start off this discussion by describing a fatal sleep disorder. If you are the type of person who will lie awake all night thinking that you have fatal familial insomnia, let me put your mind at ease. This disease is extremely rare and completely inherited; that is, you cannot acquire the disease if you don't have the gene. There are only about fifty families in the world with this genetic mutation, so if you have never heard of it, you don't have it. If you still cannot fall asleep, you're in luck, because there are many other types of insomnia that won't kill you, and the internet is full of helpful hints to improve sleep quality. Examples include the following: don't drink coffee, don't drink alcohol, don't take naps, don't go to bed at different times every night, don't eat anything after six o'clock, don't look at a screen before bed, don't do anything in your bedroom besides sleep, and don't do anything else you can possibly think of that you enjoy.

Research to support this type of advice is often done at universities, so I decided to conduct my own university research, which consisted of me sitting around and thinking back on my years at the University of Maryland. As I recall, I slept better in college than at any other time in my life. During those years, I drank coffee and/or beer any time of the day or night, took naps more often than I showered, never went to bed two nights at the same time, ate more after six o'clock than any other time of the day, fell asleep looking at a screen, and did just about everything in my bedroom.

I used advanced statistical analysis to conclude that if you want to be able to fall asleep in less than ten seconds, you have two options: go to college or have a baby. College is the cheaper option, even if you go to Harvard and pay full tuition for eight years.

If you don't happen to be a multimillionaire, there are other do-it-yourself options. One of the more creative ones I've heard came from one of my daughters, who instructed her younger sister to "tense up every muscle in your body for thirty seconds, then relax and you'll fall right to sleep." This resulted in a blood-curdling scream as she sent herself into a full body cramp. Other popular techniques include counting backward from one hundred, singing "Ninety-nine Bottles of Beer on the Wall" in your head, and the ever-popular counting sheep. As a student and a parent, I actually found these methods to be more effective for helping me to stay awake all night.

In Mitch Albom's best seller *Tuesdays with Morrie*, Morrie talks a lot about what he calls the "tension of opposites" that permeates every aspect of life. In my opinion and experience, this concept absolutely applies to sleep, in that the harder you try to fall asleep, the more awake you feel. The opposite is true as well: If you try to stay awake, you can hardly keep your eyes open. It works with almost anything. If you read that lima beans are bad for you, so you decide never to eat them again, you will spend your entire day craving lima beans. The key is to use this phenomenon to your advantage. If you can't sleep, stop trying to sleep. If you're awake at three in the morning, get up and read a book and try to stay awake. In fact, the book you are reading right now has been shown to cure many types of insomnia, so there is a good chance that you will be in a deep state of unconsciousness before you make it to the end of this chapter.

If this does not work, then you may need an evaluation by your physician. There are serious conditions that will not respond to helpful hints from me or anyone else and require actual medical treatment. Highly trained physicians often know immediately when a patient has a medical sleep disorder by the way they are still awake after sitting in the waiting room for seven hours. They may order further testing to diagnose specific problems and prescribe treatments. Do not just accept the fact that you have a hard time sleeping. Recent research shows that sleep is even more important than previously thought, and diminished quality and quantity of sleep affects virtually every aspect of mental and physical health.[1,2,3,4,5]

On the other hand, if you are able to sleep well but choose not to, you are not alone. American culture has glamorized sleep deprivation, and workaholics everywhere compete for the latest nights, hardest work schedules, and fewest days off. If you fall into this category, I recommend that you make an appointment to see me as soon as possible so I can give you a dope slap. Voluntary, chronic, enthusiastic, boastful sleep deprivation contributes to early death from many causes, including diabetes, heart disease, stroke, obesity, cancer, and degenerative neurological diseases such as Alzheimer's.[6,7,8,9,10]

I know that many of you short-sleep enthusiasts are not deterred by news reports of the above risks. So in an effort to scare the crap out of you, I will briefly describe in a little more detail the relationship between sleep and two conditions that many people believe they have little control over: Alzheimer's disease and cancer.

Alzheimer's disease attacks specific areas of the brain, including the prefrontal cortex, where executive functions such as planning, decision-making, and problem solving are performed. The prefrontal cortex also generates the brain waves that produce the deepest stages of sleep, when short-term memories are converted to long-term memories.

Alzheimer's disease deprives its victims of deep sleep. "Sticky clumps" of a protein called beta-amyloid accumulate in the prefrontal cortex and block the generation of brain waves that trigger deep sleep, thus blocking the conversion of short-term memories to long-term memories.

But this is only half of the story, because this cause and effect goes the other way as well; that is, chronic sleep deprivation can increase the risk of Alzheimer's disease because of something called the glymphatic system.

The glymphatic system in the brain is similar to the lymphatic system in the rest of the body. The lymphatic system is a network of ducts and vessels that carry a clear liquid called lymph. This fluid delivers white blood cells to the body's tissues to fight infection and carries toxins and waste products away from these tissues. In a similar fashion, the glymphatic system carries waste products, including excess beta-amyloid, out of the brain. This glymphatic system is ten to twenty times more active during the deepest stages of sleep. So if you chronically deprive yourself of sufficient durations of deep sleep, your glymphatic system will not have time to sufficiently clear these waste products from your brain. Not surprisingly, studies have shown a higher risk of Alzheimer's disease in people who are chronically sleep-deprived.[11]

As for cancer, research shows that one of the most powerful forces in cancer prevention is the immune system.[12] Natural "killer cells" that circulate through your bloodstream constantly round up and destroy cells that would otherwise grow into cancer. Sleep deprivation can have a devastating effect on your immune system. One study showed that a single night of four hours of sleep destroyed 70 percent of the natural killer cells in circulation, and another showed a 40 percent increase in cancer risk for those who are chronically sleep-deprived.[13]

The problem is that everyone knows someone who claims to need only four hours of sleep per night, and the thought of this is enticing. Just think of how much you could get done, or how much extra time you would have to enjoy the things you like to do. There are never enough hours in a day. Four extra hours each day translates to twenty-eight hours each week—more than a full extra day. If time is money, this would truly be a windfall.

In an effort to cash in on this concept, many people, myself included, have tried to train themselves to require less sleep. I couldn't do it. No matter how disciplined and gradual I was with my program, the weariness, fatigue, and downright exhaustion would eventually become unbearable. I now know the reason for this: The amount of sleep you need is genetic. There are those who only need four hours per night, but the reason is that they have an extremely rare mutation on a gene called DEC2.[14] People with this mutation do not need to train themselves to be short-sleepers; they simply wake up refreshed and alert with no urge to stay in bed and suffer no adverse health effects.

It has been estimated that fewer than one in twelve thousand people have this gene mutation.[15] Interestingly, and perhaps as a result of our cultural admiration for short-sleepers, up to 99 percent of short-sleepers who believe they have this mutation actually do not—and end up suffering many long term health consequences. The vast majority of people are genetically wired to need about seven to eight hours of sleep per night.

Several other aspects of sleep turn out to be genetic as well, such as how your body processes and reacts to caffeine[16] and whether you are a "morning person" or a "night owl."[17] So don't beat yourself up trying to be something you're not. Sleep is a hardwired function that is absolutely necessary for good health and normal life span.

I could not end this discussion without mentioning one of my favorite aspects of sleep: the power nap. I perfected the power nap in college. I could sit in a lecture hall with my head perfectly balanced over my shoulders and fall sound asleep without moving. Less experienced nappers would jerk themselves awake and fall into the aisles, but not me. To this day, I can sleep anywhere. If I get tired driving, I pull over and close my eyes for exactly ten minutes (as I mentioned before, do not do this at red lights—it is extremely dangerous) and wake up completely refreshed. I once took a nap standing up on a bus.

Years later I was thrilled to find out that research had validated my long-held belief in the benefits of power naps. Short bursts of sleep decrease levels of adenosine, which is a chemical that builds up in your brain while you are awake and makes you feel drowsy. In fact, adenosine levels play a large role in regulating our natural sleep-wake cycles.[18]

Most humans are monophasic sleepers—that is, they sleep once per twenty-four-hour day for a relatively long period of time. It turns out that the vast majority of mammals are biphasic or polyphasic sleepers, sleeping for shorter durations two or more times per day.[19] Some researchers now believe that social forces have forced humans into monophasic sleep patterns, and that we are naturally wired to be biphasic sleepers. In fact, research has revealed lower mortality rates from conditions such as heart disease in cultures where siestas—or short midday naps—are the norm.[20] So here is my advice to all you workaholics: Take a real lunch break, go out to your car, recline the seat, close your eyes, and sleep for ten minutes. And if you get in trouble, tell your boss I said it was okay.

5

STRENGTHENING

As a young boy I discovered the benefits of weight training and in a few short months was able to transform myself from a skinny, awkward kid into a skinny, awkward kid with tendinitis. Now, as a professional physical therapist, I draw on this experience to teach my patients how to train with weights correctly. Strength training can cause a lot of damage if done incorrectly. I've treated scores of patients whose response, when I asked them how they got hurt, started with, "Well, I was lifting weights and . . ."

The most important thing to remember when weight training is to maintain good form. I learned long ago that whether I'm treating a seasoned gym rat or a lifelong couch potato, I need to keep a close eye on my patients as they do their exercises, no matter how long they have been coming to therapy. It is very easy to let your mind wander and lose concentration while exercising. I have had patients who demonstrate perfect form for weeks, and I turn my head for a few seconds and look back to see them performing what looks like the chicken dance. Good form is essential for injury prevention, so remember to perform your exercises slowly, keep your stomach muscles tight, use weights you can handle, and don't use momentum to swing the weights. If you are not working with a therapist or trainer, exercise with a partner so you can keep an eye on each other's form.

The past few years have seen a rise in popularity of home work-out routines with names like P90X, P90Xtralarge, Insanity, Insanity II, Insanity for the Completely Insane, and Insanity for Sociopaths. These training programs utilize fast, explosive motions at high intensity, and are based on the theory that flabby, middle-aged office workers are physically qualified to follow the same training regimen as the United States Marine Corps.

Gyms with names like CrossFit and Boot Camp have followed suit, with people climbing on obstacles and flailing around with ropes. When I was a teenager, the most complex exercise at my gym was called "squat," so we have definitely come a long way. As someone who makes a living off of other people's injuries, I would like to officially recommend these programs as a great way to improve my salary. For you old-schoolers out there who want nothing to do with these newfangled routines, I would highly recommend that you catch up with the times. I have a boat payment due.

For those who are not interested in paying for my boat, you may want to stay away from these programs, at least in the early stages of your training. Slow, controlled motions are still the safest way to train for strength, especially for beginners.

Many people lift weights to get big and strong, which is fine, but that is not what this book is about. Rather, this chapter will explain how to lift weights to rehabilitate injuries and to improve health and well-being. When these are the goals, there are three main reasons to exercise with weights: to increase circulation, to protect the joints, and to improve movement patterns. Let's look at these one at a time, starting with circulation. I will repeat this concept over and over: It all comes down to circulation. Blood is the key. It carries everything to the tissues of your body. Oxygen, nutrients, protein, minerals, vitamins, immune cells, hormones, and everything else you need to live are transported to your body's tissues by blood. Strengthening exercises dramatically increase blood flow because muscles have a great blood supply. They are packed with blood vessels, and when you lift weights these blood vessels dilate and circulation increases to about twenty times resting rate.[1] Your heart also beats stronger and faster during exercise, so your bloodstream literally forces oxygen and nutrients into the tissues of your body.

The second reason to exercise with weights is to protect the joints. This may seem counterintuitive. You may think that weightlifting increases the stress on joints and contributes to more wear and tear. This is true if you lift incorrectly with weights that are too heavy. You will notice that "to be able to lift a car" is not on my list of reasons to exercise with weights. Proper lifting technique with moderate weight strengthens muscles without damaging joints. These muscles protect the joints by absorbing your body weight. If your muscles become weak, they absorb less force, and the burden of bearing your body weight shifts directly to the joints and causes more wear and tear.

The third reason to exercise with weights is to improve movement patterns. This is accomplished by "waking up" certain muscle groups. Many people develop pain because they do not contract the right muscles at the right times when they move. If you have ever watched shows like *The Biggest Loser*, you have heard trainers yell the popular phrase, "Fire your glutes." This technique is a very effective way to give clients something to think about besides chocolate cake. It also, at times, actually causes people to fire, or contract, their glutes, although the effectiveness of this maneuver depends on their understanding of what this actually means. (I had one patient turn, look at her butt, and say, "You're fired!")

I will discuss this concept in more detail later when I talk about injuries, but for now I will just mention that there are ways to facilitate proper muscle contraction without yelling at your body parts. For example, I have treated patients who have sharp pain in the front of their knees when they try to step up onto a six-inch box. I put a resistance stretch band around their ankles and instruct them to sidestep back and forth across the room a few times. Then they step up on the box again, and the pain is gone. What happened? Before performing the sidestepping exercise, the muscles on the sides of their hips were not firing properly. When muscles don't do their job, other muscles try to pick up the slack and fire too much, which causes too much force in one area, causing pain. The muscles on the sides of the hips do not get stronger after just doing a few side steps. They are just "woken up." The sidestepping motion forces these muscles to contract, and that contraction carries over to the next activity. This is a more effective way to get specific muscles to fire than by just saying, "Concentrate on contracting the muscles on the side of your hips." A good workout routine should include exercises that force commonly underused muscles to wake up.

Again, I will get into more detail with these types of exercises later. For now, I will define "strength" and describe the basics of how to strengthen weak muscles. If you are familiar with weight training, you may already know much of what I am about to say, so forgive me if it seems simplistic. The following story illustrates the reason why I do not want to assume that you already know these basics.

While covering for another therapist one day, I was treating a patient who'd had a total knee replacement about three months prior. Since her surgery she had been coming to therapy three times per week doing nothing but exercises to get her leg stronger. By this time she was so familiar with her exercises that she could practically do them in her sleep. I happened to be treating her on her last day of therapy, and toward the end of the session she looked at me and asked, in all seriousness, "Before I get discharged I wanted to ask you, are there any exercises I can do to get my leg stronger?"

Well yes, actually, you know all of those exercises you have been doing for the last three months? They were all specifically designed to get your leg stronger. This was breaking news. Her treating therapist evidently forgot to mention this. It's not just doctors who rush in and out of rooms without explaining anything. At least they have the somewhat valid reason that three nanoseconds is physically not enough time to explain much. But this physical therapist saw this lady for an hour, three times a week, *for three months.*

So to avoid repeating this mistake, I will now explain the basics. Strength is the ability of a muscle to contract and generate force. There are three types of muscle contractions: concentric, eccentric, and isometric.

A concentric contraction causes movement in the same direction as the contraction. When you lift a box from the floor to a table, you are pulling up and the box is moving up, so this is a concentric activity.

An eccentric contraction causes movement in the opposite direction as the contraction. When you slowly lower a heavy box to the floor, you are pulling up to control the motion, but the box is moving down, so this is an eccentric activity.

An isometric contraction stabilizes but causes no movement. When you stand and hold a box without moving, your muscles are contracting to prevent you and the box from falling to the floor, but there is no motion, so this is an isometric activity.

There are also different types of muscle fibers that exhibit different types of strength. The two main types are fast-twitch and slow-twitch. Fast-twitch muscles generate high forces at high speeds, but they have poor endurance and run out of gas quickly. Slow-twitch muscles generate lower forces at lower speeds, but they have great endurance and can continue contracting for long periods of time. Most muscles contain both types of fibers in varying proportions. Some muscles contain mostly slow-twitch, others mostly fast-twitch.

Muscle physiology can get complicated, but you do not have to get lost in the technical weeds in order to understand the basics of strength: three types of contractions (concentric, eccentric, and isometric), and two types of muscles (fast-twitch and slow-twitch). If you remember these basics, then you will understand the most important feature of strength training: *specificity*.

Muscles respond to the demands placed on them. If muscles consistently work hard, they get stronger. If they do very little work, they get weaker. But strengthening is a bit more complicated than that because of specificity: To train muscles for a fast, explosive activity such as a hundred-meter dash, fast, explosive exercises must be done; to train for a long, slow endurance event such as a marathon, long-duration exercises must be done.

Someone once asked me why a large, muscular powerlifter can't throw a baseball faster than a thin major-league pitcher, since the powerlifter is obviously stronger. The answer is that while the powerlifter's muscles can contract with more force, the pitcher's muscles can contract with more speed, which is more important when moving a light object as fast as possible. The training is specific to the task.

Genetics play a large role as well. Some people are born with more fast-twitch muscles and are better suited to fast, explosive activities. And those born with more slow-twitch muscles will have better natural endurance. Training can make a difference, but everyone has their own physiological limit for any particular activity. A world-class marathon runner can improve sprinting speed with training but will never transform into a world-class sprinter.

I use these athletic examples to illustrate the concepts of strength training, but what do these mean for average people who just want to stay healthy? First, if you fall into this category, I don't want you to worry about fast-twitch and slow-twitch. Fast, ballistic exercises carry increased risks of injuries, and only athletes who have gradually worked up to this level of training should perform them. I do, however, want you to be aware of the three types of contractions—concentric, eccentric, and isometric—because everyday activities continually employ all three. And if you exercise with slow, controlled motions, you will train all three types of movements: slow on the way up (concentric), brief pause at the top (isometric), and slow on the way down (eccentric).

It is impossible to describe a strength training routine that is appropriate for everyone reading this book. A forty-five-year-old office worker should have a different regimen than a twenty-two-year-old bartender. And someone who wants to lift weights for an hour every day will perform a different routine than someone who can only spare twenty minutes twice a week. There are thousands of exercises, and the possible combinations of workout routines are almost endless. There are many books, magazines, and websites available to help you design a program, so I will not get into those details here. What I will do is describe three basic rules you should follow for any level of strength training.

Rule #1: Work muscle groups on both sides of every joint.

This means that for every "pulling" exercise, you should have a "pushing" exercise. This will prevent muscles on one side of a joint from becoming stronger than those on the other side. A muscle imbalance increases the chance of injury because the weaker side of the joint cannot stand up to the forces generated by the stronger side.

Rule #2: Never work the same body part two days in a row.

Strength training actually breaks down muscle tissues. This improves strength because when you rest, your body builds these tissues back up stronger than they were before. If you train the same muscles on consecutive days, you further break down the tissues before the body has a chance to build them back up. If you work the same body part every day, you will continue to break down the muscle tissues to the point of injury, and you will lose strength.

This rule only applies to heavy lifting, which means using weights that make it impossible to perform more than fifteen repetitions in a row and performing multiple sets of each exercise to failure. Physical therapists often prescribe light lifting exercises to rehabilitate injuries, and these can be done every day. Exercise routines utilizing light weights with a high number of repetitions can also be done on consecutive days.

You can perform heavy lifting every day as long as you don't work the same body parts for two days in a row. Mix up your workouts by training different body parts on different days.

Rule #3: Don't forget about the rest days.

This applies to all exercise regimens, not just weight training. As mentioned above in rule number two, your body actually builds itself up and gets stronger during rest. So not only should you alternate workouts to rest different body parts on different days, but you should also include days of total rest so that all of the body's systems have a chance to recover. Rest days are so important that I once designed a workout routine that consisted of only rest days. (This didn't actually work that well.)

These three basic rules will help the average person design a safe program. But since many of you are not average, I feel the need to speak to those on the ends of the spectrum. So let me start with those of you who have never lifted weights and want nothing to do with lifting weights. I know you are out there, because I have met many of you. You are in this category if you firmly believe the following:

1. Going to a gym is the single biggest waste of time in the history of the universe.
2. You get plenty of exercise by getting things done (vacuuming, cutting grass, etc.) or by going for walks.
3. There is no such thing as "good pain."

If these statements sum up your position, you are not alone, and I am painfully aware of the enormity of my chosen task, which is to convince you to give weightlifting a try. So let's address your beliefs, starting with the gym. "How can you spend all that time and energy and get nothing done?" I've heard it a million times, and I honestly understand the point. When I was young and single, I felt very productive lifting weights at the gym. But when I reached that stage of life when I had to work twelve hours per day, sleep four hours per night, fix everything that broke around the house, and somehow find time to feed, bathe, clothe, and entertain babies and toddlers, the thought of going to the gym seemed like the most ridiculous waste of time imaginable. So I do understand that line of thinking. Many people feel much more productive getting a workout by getting things done. And some people just find exercise incredibly boring.

But here's the thing. Vacuuming and cutting grass are good exercises, but they are not the same as strength training because they do not involve repetitions to fatigue. Performing a motion against resistance until you can't do any more, resting, and then repeating this several times opens more capillaries and fills the muscles with more blood than performing even fairly strenuous activities like cutting grass. If you try this type of workout you will immediately feel the difference, and over time you will gain much more strength.

And what about walking? It is great exercise, don't get me wrong. Don't stop walking. But if walking is your only exercise, you could actually be at risk for injury, because walking is a repetitive motion activity. You repeat the same motion over and over thousands of times, and this can cause wear and tear and lead to painful inflammation. Repetitive motion injury is a medical diagnosis for which I get referrals all the time. And walking does nothing for flexibility because you don't need to move your legs very far to take a step. I have treated hundreds of avid walkers who are extremely tight.

So what I'd like to do is make a deal with you. I will bet that if you give it a try, you will discover that the benefits of strength training are so enormous that when you feel what they do for your body, you will wish that you had been lifting weights all your life. You may even begin to understand that phrase, "It hurts but it feels good." Before you say no, let me just add that you will not need to go anywhere near a gym or put on anything that resembles yoga pants. And wait, there's more. I can outline a program that will take only fifteen minutes, twice per week, and provide you with tremendous benefits. If you are willing to give this a try, you will find this program in appendix I, "Strength Training for Those Who Hate Exercise."

Now for those of you at the other end of the spectrum. You are in this category if you have ever done one of the following:

1. Flexed your muscles in front of a mirror in a crowded gym where everyone can see you.
2. Trapped yourself under a barbell in your basement trying to bench press double your body weight.
3. Known your bicep measurement off the top of your head.

If you are in this group, I want to personally thank you for the years of guaranteed income you have provided for me and my family. At the risk of losing some of this revenue, I'm going to let you in on a secret that some of my older patients have told me: Very heavy weight-lifting is not worth it. When you are young it feels great, and you really do believe you are doing the right thing for your body. But over the years, heavy lifting takes a toll on your joints that can ruin the last third of your life. I have had men and women, some as young as fifty, say to me, "I thought I was invincible; I don't know what I was thinking." If you are a competitive lifter, I know I am not going to talk you out of heavy lifting. But as you age, your quality of life will improve greatly if you cross-train, stretch, decrease weights, increase reps, and get plenty of rest days. And your joints will thank you even more if you start these habits when you are young.

I'm all for a good, hard workout, but there is a difference between pushing yourself to the limit and being ridiculous. I've seen people pass out and I've seen tendons tear right off bones. It's not good for you. Even professional football players talk about the difference between "weight room strength" and "grown-man strength." The guy with weight room strength can lift more weight than you, but the guy with grown-man strength can use technique and leverage to control you out on the football field, and that is much more important. Use good form with weights you can handle and your body will serve you well into old age. If not, you may need a walker when you're fifty.

6

STRETCHING

Humans first discovered the benefits of stretching during medieval times. They even built elaborate machines with affectionate names like "the rack" to loosen people up so they would admit things that they otherwise would not. In a similar fashion, modern physical therapists use manual stretching techniques to motivate uncooperative patients who are reluctant to cough up their copays.

But the benefits of stretching do not end there. Stretching is one of the best things you can do for your body, whether you are injured or healthy, because it improves flexibility and decreases the soft tissue tightness that causes many everyday aches and pains. And you do not need to turn yourself into a contortionist in order to benefit from stretching. Even small gains in flexibility translate into substantial improvements in how you feel. In fact, the amount of flexibility you gain is largely dependent on your genetic makeup. Structural proteins called collagen and elastin are the primary building blocks of soft tissues. There are many types of collagen, but type I and type III are found in muscles, tendons, and ligaments. Type I collagen is quite stiff, whereas type III collagen is more flexible. Elastin is also very flexible. The ratio of these three proteins determines your genetic flexibility. People with high percentages of elastin and type III collagen are naturally flexible, while those who have mostly type I collagen are naturally tight and can gain only limited amounts of measurable flexibility by stretching. So it is important not to compare yourself to others, especially in a busy clinic or crowded gym.

Many patients say to me, "I've never had good flexibility." If this is something you would say, it is even more important for you to stretch, for several reasons. First, even if you feel like you are getting nowhere, stretching is likely preventing you from becoming even tighter than you already are. We all know the average eighty-year-old is not as flexible as the average twenty-year-old. This loss of flexibility happens gradually over the life span, and stretching can significantly slow down this process. I have treated middle-aged and older patients who gained relatively small amounts of measurable flexibility but returned months later to tell me that they kept up with their stretching programs because they significantly decreased their aches and pains.

Second, stretching has been shown to induce stem cells to differentiate into soft tissue components such as the above-mentioned collagen and elastin, which means that it stimulates your body to produce more of the elastic materials that make up your soft tissues.[1]

And third, research has shown that stretching increases blood flow and angiogenesis (the formation of new blood vessels),[2] which is great for all of the body's tissues. Improved circulation decreases the chance of injuries and improves healing when injuries do occur.

There are certain groups of people who, generally, hate to stretch, among them long-distance runners. The reason most give is that running takes so much time, they don't want to spend more time doing anything else. But I have seen many of these endurance athletes grow to love stretching. I once treated a world-class Iron Man triathlete who spent several months rehabilitating an ankle injury. He had poor flexibility in all of his leg muscles, so I initiated a comprehensive stretching program. At first he wanted nothing to do with this, but by the end of his course of rehab he would preach the benefits of stretching to all of the other patients in the clinic and describe in detail how stretching took minutes off his running times.

TYPES OF STRETCHING

There are several different types of stretching, but I will describe the three main types that I use: static stretching, dynamic stretching, and active stretching.

Static Stretching

A static stretch is held for a sustained period of time—usually ten to twenty seconds—without bouncing or moving. This is typically repeated five to ten times, with a one- to two-second rest in between. The body part being stretched must be relaxed while a force is applied to move it to the end range. You can apply this force yourself by pulling on the limb or leaning into a stationary object. If someone else applies this force, it is called manual stretching.

Manual stretching can produce better results in some patients because they can more easily relax when they are not trying to simultaneously pull. However, the opposite effect sometimes occurs when things like apprehension, pain, or fear cause patients to reflexively resist and stiffen.

Some research on static stretching has caused controversy in recent years. Studies show that static stretching done just before activity can actually have a detrimental effect on athletic performance, and some trainers and sports teams have gone so far as to abandon static stretching as a matter of protocol.[3,4] Other research, however, shows that if it is not done right before the measured athletic activity, a regular program of static stretching increases muscle length by increasing the number of sarcomeres (the microscopic units of muscle tissue)[5] and actually improves athletic performance in the long term.[6]

If done the right way at the right time, static stretching is beneficial. It should not be done first thing in the morning or right before activity, especially fast, ballistic activity such as sprinting. The best time is at the end of a workout or after a warm-up activity such as a brisk walk or a stationary-bike ride. Static stretching should be done gently and should not produce a sharp, severe pain, but rather a good stretching sensation in the right place. (When I describe how to rehabilitate specific injuries, I will tell you where the right places are.)

There are times when aggressive static stretching is needed to treat certain medical conditions, which I will discuss in more detail in chapter 16. This type of stretching should be done only under the supervision of a physical therapist.

Dynamic Stretching

Athletes often use dynamic stretching techniques, which involve swinging motions that take a joint to its limit at each end of the swing. These faster motions are not quite as safe as slower, more controlled techniques and can cause injuries if done too aggressively. But if done correctly and carefully, they are safe for just about anyone. The key is to start with slow, short swings, build up slowly, and don't go past the point of comfort. Unlike static stretching, dynamic stretching is a good way to start a workout and can serve as a good warm-up before athletic activities such as sprinting or jumping.

Active Stretching

When you get out of bed and stretch your arms over your head, you perform an active stretch. This type of stretch moves a joint to the end-range of motion using the joint's own muscle contraction, as opposed to you or someone else applying overpressure. An active stretch is one of the best ways to treat a new injury because it generates less force than a static stretch and it is slower and more controlled than a dynamic stretch.

GENERAL TIPS FOR STRETCHING

You can stretch every day or even twice per day if you like. But it is wise to take a day off every so often to allow recovery. How far you can stretch will vary from day to day. Your body is not a static machine; it is a living organism that is in a constant state of change. Diet, fluid intake, sleep, mood, rest, and the constant ebb and flow of body chemistry all factor into your flexibility. You may feel very tight one day, and loose and flexible the next. This is normal. Alter the intensity of your stretching based on how you feel. If you feel tight, stretch more gently. If you feel tight for several days in a row, take a day off. If you hear a loud snapping noise and feel sharp, excruciating pain, you probably pushed too hard.

7

ENDURANCE TRAINING

All of my patients are referred by a physician. I previously described what patients have to go through to actually see a physician, and I know that if they made it through this process, they already have superhuman endurance. So that's one less thing I have to worry about. For those of you who have tried to see a physician and just not made it, keep trying. Many marathon runners didn't make it on their first or even second attempts. My advice is, be prepared. I have a doctor's appointment in three months, and I've already started carb loading.

Endurance is critical not only for surviving doctors' appointments but for the survival of the entire human species, from prehistoric humans who had to walk miles to find food and water, to modern humans who have to make it from their cubicles to the vending machine several times every day. When you look at it this way, it is obvious that life itself is an endurance event. In addition to the normal demands of everyday life, modern humans have also figured out how to simulate the activities of their prehistoric ancestors with high-tech equipment. Some examples of these are the elliptical trainer, which simulates searching for food and water on an elliptical trainer, and the stair-stepper, which simulates searching for food and water on a stair-stepper.

There are several important reasons to incorporate endurance training into your routine. First, if you want to burn off fat, endurance training is the only way to do it. Lifting weights will not burn off fat at specific areas of your body. Working the muscles on the back of your arms will not burn off those bags of flab on the back of your arms, and sit-ups will not burn the fat off your stomach. This is because your body burns through other sources of energy before it burns fat, and this does not start to happen until your heart rate is elevated for about twenty to thirty minutes. Furthermore, once you do start burning fat, there is no way to tell your body where to burn it off first. Your body burns it wherever it decides to burn it. Lifting weights strengthens and tones the muscles that are buried underneath the fat, but it does not burn off the fat.

Second—here we go again—the all-important circulation: Endurance training improves the circulation in your cardiovascular system, which consists of your heart, lungs, and blood vessels. When you run, walk, swim, bike, or do anything physical for a sustained period of time (twenty minutes or more), your heart becomes stronger and more efficient, your lungs expand and increase the amount of oxygen they can transfer to the blood, your blood vessels widen, and new blood vessels grow, like branches of a tree, in response to your body's need for more oxygen. This is why physicians prescribe endurance exercises for patients with circulation problems. Weight training and stretching alone do not adequately improve cardiovascular endurance and circulation. I have seen bodybuilders with huge muscles become short of breath walking up one flight of stairs.

Having said that, there are ways to lift weights to improve endurance. If you cut back the weights to moderate levels, perform several exercises in succession without rest in between, and repeat this cycle several times, you will get an excellent cardiovascular workout. Wrestlers and other athletes who require high levels of endurance often perform this type of workout, which is called circuit training.

Fast walking, running, cycling, swimming, and working out on machines like the aforementioned elliptical trainer and stair-stepper are all great ways to develop endurance. The intensity depends on your level of fitness and available time. If you read something like, "Exercising on a treadmill burns more calories than exercising on a bike," don't take it too seriously, and don't feel like you need to run out and spend money on that particular piece of equipment. The amount of calories you burn depends on the intensity and length of time of your workout, not the apparatus. The machine does not get you in shape; you get yourself in shape on the machine.

The most important recommendation I have when it comes to endurance training is to cross-train, which means mixing up your workouts and performing different routines on different days. I am a strong believer in cross-training for many types of exercise, but particularly for endurance training, because endurance activities involve repetitive motions. When you walk, run, swim, bike, or work out on a machine for long periods of time, you perform the same motions over and over, and this can cause repetitive motion injuries. If you are a creature of habit, you don't have to do a different workout every day, but you should change it up at least once a month.

And remember, no amount of exercise is a waste of time. People have busy and logistically complicated lives. If you can only find a little time to exercise, then do it! I don't care if your only workout is taking the stairs instead of the elevator. If you think this has no benefit, then you have an excuse to do nothing. Every bit of exercise makes a positive difference.

8

THE AGING BODY

You know you're getting old when your face doesn't look exactly like it did when you were sixteen. If you are unlucky enough to suffer from this debilitating condition, there is hope. Thanks to painful and expensive surgical procedures, your aging face can be transformed into an aging face that looks like it was inflated like a party balloon.

If you happen to have some sort of squeamish aversion to surgery, that doesn't mean you have to surrender to the effects of aging. Thanks to modern pharmaceuticals, there are drugs that can do just about anything to keep you looking and feeling young. All you need is expensive insurance and enough money left over to afford the out-of-pocket costs, and these easy-to-swallow pills can lower your blood pressure, increase your energy level, lower your cholesterol, control your diabetes, and, if you're lucky enough to be a man way past normal reproductive age, give you an erection you could hang a stepladder on.

If you're on a tight budget, or just want to stay youthful without surgery or chemicals, there is a way to do that too: proper diet, sleep, and exercise. (Sound familiar?) If you are diligent about these things, you will be able to easily keep up with the younger folks. Ever finish a meal and the kids all pop up and bounce away like it was the easiest thing in the world, while you struggle to get your creaky bones moving? Well, no more! If you follow this plan, those kids will struggle to keep up with you.

I was lucky enough to learn at an early age that if I kept myself fit and ate a healthy diet, I could completely avoid all those pitfalls of aging, like losing my eyesight and being stiff and sore all the time. So I did everything right, and now that I am in my fifties, I am losing my eyesight and I am stiff and sore all the time.

What happened? I'll tell you what happened. When I was young I had the same delusion that my kids have now when they make fun of the way I search around for my reading glasses and inform me that they will never get to the point of doing something so ridiculous even if they live to be 150, which they fully believe they will. That's the thing I miss most about youth: the sincere and honest belief that I was completely different from every single one of the trillions of mammals that have lived, gotten old, and died on this planet.

So let me lay down a little reality: Even if you do everything right, you are still going to age. You will be more stiff and sore than when you were young. If you are lucky enough to live a long life, you will reach a point when things will start to decline, including your eyesight, hearing, strength, memory, and fashion sense. It's just life. The good news is, if you are diligent about proper diet, sleep, and exercise, you will likely fare much better and enjoy your life more than if you passively let the aging process unfold. And you will have a lower chance of suffering from serious health problems. No guarantees. You are just playing the odds.

I wanted to get that off my chest so I don't get irate letters from eighty-five-year-olds who are angry at me because they followed my advice and still can't do back handsprings.

I realize that in our culture, it is hard to admit that you shouldn't try back handsprings when you are eighty-five. Just look at our role models. In 2014, George H. W. Bush jumped out of a perfectly good airplane on his ninetieth birthday. In 1975, at age sixty-one, famous fitness expert Jack LaLanne put on scuba gear and swam the length of the Golden Gate Bridge, underwater, hands and feet bound, while towing a one-thousand-pound boat. And in 2017, at the age of eighty-eight, Betty Bromage became the oldest female wing walker in the UK. These and other inspiring stories show that you are never too old to develop the wisdom and good judgment of a twelve-year-old. I'm all for a good time and a little adventure, but the average person cannot perform the above activities and walk away unscathed. Personally, if I make it to ninety, I plan on celebrating the event by flying across the country without jumping out of the airplane.

You need to use your brain more as you age. You need to pay more attention to how things feel. Is that a good pain or a bad pain?

Should you change up your workout routine here, or add another rest day there? Thought and judgment become more important. If you spent years pushing through pain and bouncing back from injuries in your youth, the need to set reasonable limits can be frustrating. But overcoming that challenge and figuring out exactly what works for your body can also be very rewarding. If you push through pain as you get older, you run a higher risk of permanent damage. So use your brain. Be smart. And if you just can't bring yourself to do that, I want to personally thank you for putting my kids through college. I'll see you in the office.

PART III

THE INJURED BODY

9

TYPES OF INJURIES

A few years ago I took my car to the dealer for routine service. After a few hours, my mechanic called to say that after the rough winter we just had, my sway bar bushings were shot and they needed to be replaced or my axle could fall off and I could die and it would be $900. So I said go ahead and replace them because God knows I can't be driving around with worn-out sway bar bushings and I certainly don't want to die. I said this knowing full well that I had no idea what a sway bar bushing was, and he could have been selling me a $900 sun visor. But there was no way I could admit this to anyone in the automotive field.

I relate this story because many patients have the same fear of looking dumb in front of the doctor, and this fear prevents them from asking simple questions. Patients ask me, usually in a whisper, questions like, "My doctor says I have a sprain; what exactly is a sprain?" So this chapter provides quick, basic descriptions of the most common injuries and conditions.

An injury can occur with or without trauma. A traumatic injury is the result of a specific event, such as a fall or a car accident. A nontraumatic injury can come on suddenly or gradually for no apparent reason. I frequently hear, "The doctor says I have a large tear, but nothing happened so how can I have a tear?" It is important to understand that even a large tear in soft tissue can develop slowly over time with no sudden trauma. Think of a rope that continually rubs against the corner of a concrete wall. Over time the rope will fray, and at some point it will eventually tear.

SPRAIN/STRAIN

A tear in soft tissue is called a sprain or strain. A sprain is a tear in a ligament or joint capsule, and a strain is a tear in a muscle. They are classified by severity. Grade I is a microtear, which is a tear so small that it could only be seen under a microscope; grade II is a partial tear, big enough to be seen with the naked eye; and grade III is a complete tear.

ROTATOR CUFF TEAR

The rotator cuff is made up of four muscles that run along the shoulder blade and attach to the top of the arm bone. These deep muscles are buried beneath the large outer muscles that you can see. A rotator cuff tear is simply a tear in one or more of these muscles. This may be a small partial tear, or a large tear that completely separates the muscle from the bone.

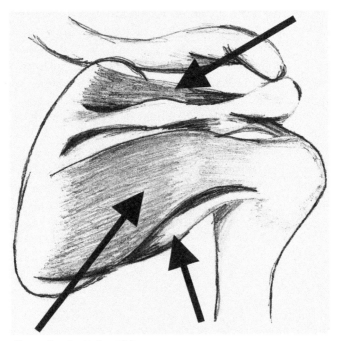

Illustration by Haley Risi

FROZEN SHOULDER

A frozen shoulder has nothing to do with being cold; it has to do with being tight. The medical term for a frozen shoulder is adhesive capsulitis. "Adhesive" means stuck together, "capsule" refers to the joint capsule, and "itis" means inflammation, so a frozen shoulder is one that is tight because the joint capsule is inflamed. This condition can occur after an injury or surgery, but commonly comes out of nowhere for no apparent reason. I talk much more about frozen shoulders in chapters 11 and 20.

IMPINGEMENT

Impingement occurs when soft tissue is pinched or squeezed between bones. This happens in many joints, but most commonly in the shoulder and hip. Impingement is caused by swelling of the soft tissue, thickening or spurring of the bones caused by calcification, or both.

DISC BULGE OR HERNIATION

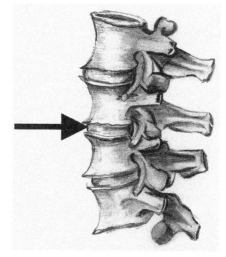

The discs between each spinal vertebra support compressive load. A bulge in the tough outer covering of the disc can develop the same way it does on a weak spot on a worn-out tire. A herniation forms if the outer covering tears and some of the gelatinous center oozes out. A bulge or herniation can cause neck or back pain. If a bulge or herniation presses on a nerve it can cause pain to shoot down the arm or leg.

The term "slipped disc" is an outdated term for a bulge or

Illustration by Haley Risi

herniation. It is a misnomer because the discs are firmly attached to the vertebrae above and below, and they don't "slip out."

PINCHED NERVE

The term "pinched nerve" is also often a misnomer. A nerve can be pinched, but it can also be compressed, squeezed, stuck down by scar tissue, under tension, swollen, or inflamed. Some clinicians use the term "pinched nerve" to describe all of these conditions, but I prefer the term "nerve irritation" to describe anything that puts abnormal force or tension on a nerve.

As a nerve courses through the body, it is tightly packed between many structures, including ligaments, muscles, tendons, discs, and bones. Any inflammation or tightness along this course can squeeze or compress a nerve and cause irritation.

Nerve irritation can cause a variety of symptoms including numbness, tingling, hot or cold sensations, sharp or dull pain, and "electric shocks." These symptoms can travel the entire length of the nerve.

TORN MENISCUS

The meniscus is a soft pad of tissue that cushions and protects the cartilage of the knee. When doctors talk about a torn cartilage, they are usually referring to a torn meniscus. Most of the meniscus, except for the outer rim, has no blood supply and is kept alive by nutrients in the synovial fluid. However, with no blood supply, injuries will not heal. Most meniscus tears occur where there is no blood supply, so if

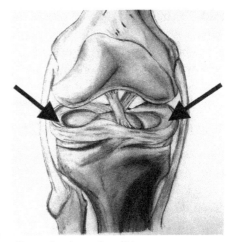

Illustration by Haley Risi

surgery is needed, the torn part is simply removed. What remains is usually sufficient to absorb body weight and protect the cartilage. Tears in the outer rim are rare and can be surgically repaired.

Not every meniscus tear requires surgery, because the pain is often the result of surrounding inflammation, not the tear itself. Many people without knee pain have meniscus tears and don't even know it. However, a large tear sometimes forms a flap that can peel up and get caught between the bones of the knee, causing sharp pain and sometimes "locking" of the joint. This is called a bucket handle tear, and almost always requires surgery.

TORN LABRUM

The hip and shoulder are ball-and-socket joints. The labrum is a rim of soft tissue that lines the socket. Like the meniscus in the knee, it protects and cushions the cartilage. Not every labral tear requires surgery, as the surrounding inflammation often causes most of the pain. But a large tear can cause locking, catching, or instability, and often requires surgery.

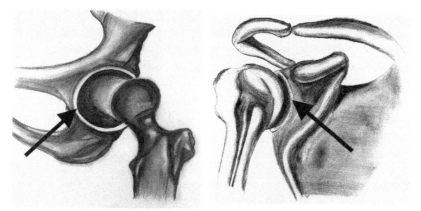

Illustrations by Haley Risi

DISLOCATION/SUBLUXATION

A dislocated joint is a joint that has popped out of position. This is very painful, and it is often necessary for a doctor to pop the joint back into place. A subluxation is a small dislocation that instantly pops back into place by itself. The terminology gets better. The process of manually popping a joint back into place is called reducing the dislocation. So if you have a dislocated finger and the doctor tells you it has to be reduced, don't worry. It doesn't mean that a surgeon is going to cut your finger off. It just means that doctors don't speak English, they speak "medical," which is a vastly complex language that was specifically designed to scare the hell out of you.

When a joint dislocates, the ligaments and joint capsule stretch beyond their normal range and become loose. This can result in an unstable joint that dislocates easily. Strengthening the surrounding muscles can help restore stability, but in severe cases surgery is needed to tighten or reconstruct the soft tissues.

BONE SPUR

A bone spur usually forms where a tendon attaches to a bone. If there is too much tension at this attachment point due to tightness or inflammation, the tendon will try to make itself stronger by absorbing calcium from the bloodstream. It actually tries to turn itself into a bone.

As a spur forms, it doesn't fully harden for weeks, so if inflammation is reduced and normal flexibility is restored before this happens, the spur may reabsorb and disappear. However, even if the spur remains, the pain may still resolve because the inflamed soft tissue around the spur usually causes most of the pain. If pain persists, a spur can be surgically removed.

PLANTAR FASCIITIS

Plantar fasciitis is an inflammation of the plantar fascia, which is a thick, tough ligament that runs from the heel to the ball of the foot. This inflammation usually develops with no traumatic injury. Tight calf muscles contribute to plantar fasciitis because they don't absorb the force of each step as well as flexible calf muscles. Force that is not absorbed by the calf travels to the bottom of the foot.

Pain from plantar fasciitis is sharp and can feel like a knife going into the heel, arch, or entire bottom of the foot. Pain typically occurs with weightbearing, especially right after prolonged sitting or lying.

ARTHRITIS

"Arthro" means joint, and "itis" means inflammation, so arthritis is inflammation of a joint. The most common form of arthritis is called osteoarthritis, which is caused by normal wear and tear as you age. Like a tire on a car, a joint is subject to friction. Even the most expensive tire wears out eventually, and every joint does the same. You will get osteoarthritis if you live long enough. Osteoarthritis cannot be cured or reversed, but its progression can be slowed down with proper stretching and strengthening, and inflammation can be managed with gentle motion, medication, and ice.

Osteoarthritis can occur in one or many joints on either side of the body in no particular pattern. Other types such as rheumatoid and psoriatic arthritis are inflammatory diseases that progressively attack all joints, usually on both sides of the body equally.

USING THIS INFORMATION

Now that you know what your diagnosis means, you are ready to learn why physical therapists do what they do to help your injury heal.

10

THE HEALING PROCESS

A patient sat on my treatment table one day and described how she injured herself. (You may recognize this patient from the introduction.) Apparently, she read in a magazine how to make homemade bath oil and decided to make some to give out as Christmas presents. She bought all the ingredients but couldn't find the specific type of oil called for in the article, so she used olive oil. She wanted to test it out before giving it to her friends and family, so she took a bath in this concoction and got so slippery that she could not get out of the bathtub. She had to call out to her husband down the hall to help her out, and during the extraction process she fell on her shoulder and he strained his back, a two-for-one deal I could not turn down.

This case highlights the most important skill that a physical therapist must cultivate: keeping a straight face. It also shows that even if you have common sense and do everything right, you can still get hurt by something as innocent as crawling into a tub of salad dressing.

After an injury like this, most people don't know what to do. I hear it every day: "I didn't know whether to move it or hold it still. Was I hurting it or helping it?" To answer these questions, you must understand different types of injuries and how they heal. The phrase "how they heal" is key, because physical therapists do not heal your injuries. Nor do chiropractors, doctors, or massage therapists. Your body heals itself, and if you understand this process, you can create the conditions that allow healing to proceed in the most efficient and effective way.

Healing is a cellular process that occurs when damaged tissue repairs itself. Healing time depends on several factors. A microinjury—one so small that it could only be seen under a microscope—may heal in a few days, although it can still be quite painful. A large tear or a broken bone can take many weeks to heal. Six weeks is considered standard healing time for this type of injury, but people who smoke, have poor circulation, or suffer from conditions like diabetes will heal more slowly.

Healing quality is just as important as healing time. Healing quality refers to how the tissue ends up after it has healed. For example, if an injured joint is held completely still throughout the healing process, it will certainly heal, but it will heal tight. If an injured muscle is not used at all, it will heal weak. If you have ever been in a cast for a couple of months, you know exactly what I am talking about. When the cast comes off, the injury has healed, but you are not at all back to normal.

So, again, physical therapists do not heal you. Physical therapists perform techniques and activities, and teach you how to perform techniques and activities, that improve healing time and quality. To do this, they work to accomplish four objectives: decrease the body's response to the injury, restore normal range of motion, restore normal strength, and restore normal movement patterns. Let's look at these one at a time.

DECREASE THE BODY'S RESPONSE

Immediately after injury, your body responds with inflammation, swelling, and protective muscle spasm. As I discussed before, these mechanisms protect you from yourself. They keep you from doing further harm to the injured area. I am often asked, "If these things are nature's way of protecting the area, why would I want to get rid of them?" This is actually a very good question. The answer is the following: These mechanisms evolved over millions of years during a period of time when humans lived out in the wilderness and had to constantly move in order to get food and, more importantly, avoid becoming food. These mechanisms worked very well in that environment because injured humans still had to move around to some extent just to stay alive. Protective mechanisms didn't prevent movement, they just made us take it down a notch so the injured area could heal. We had a clear choice: move or starve. These mechanisms don't work so well in today's environment where we still have a clear choice: move or call out to the kids from the recliner to bring another tub of onion dip.

In our cushy environment, these protective mechanisms give us an excuse to not move at all. This lack of gentle early motion can cause these mechanisms to become chronic and continue to work long after they should have subsided. When this happens, they no longer help the injured area heal. Instead, they block much-needed circulation and impede healing.

Chronic inflammation in particular can actually cause permanent tissue damage. As I touched on in chapter 1, inflammation is a series of biochemical reactions that initiate tissue repair. Normal inflammation can cause an injured body part to become hot, red, painful, or swollen. If inflammation persists longer than a few days, however, it can cause tissues to become thick and tight, and may also cause adhesions to form between tissue layers that normally glide on each other. If inflammation continues for weeks, months, or years, these tissue layers can actually grow together into a thick, dysfunctional mass.

Swelling, inflammation, and muscle spasm should start to subside in a few days. Gentle early motion is the best way to facilitate this process, as long as it is done in a way that does not cause further injury.[1] In addition to gentle early motion, physical therapists often administer a variety of treatments that fall under the category of passive modalities, such as ultrasound, electric stimulation, ice, and heat. These modalities are passive because the patients do not have to do anything. They just sit there while the modalities are applied. The problem with these modalities is that they feel good and they are easier than exercises, so they make it tempting to buy into the idea that rehabilitation requires no effort. In my opinion, physical therapists who overuse passive modalities feed into this belief and do their patients a disservice. When used appropriately, passive modalities are helpful in certain situations, but they do nothing to restore normal strength, range of motion, or movement patterns. I use them sparingly, and I tell patients that these modalities are just meant to take the edge off, and by themselves they do nothing to rehabilitate their injuries.

Many physical therapists also perform manual therapy techniques, which include hands-on treatments such as deep tissue massage and joint manipulation. When used appropriately, manual therapy can be effective. But as with passive modalities, if manual techniques are overused, or used in place of active techniques, patients can fall into the trap of wanting to "just lie down on the table and have someone work on me."

For most injuries, gentle early motion in combination with ice or heat is sufficient to keep the body's responses from spiraling out of control. If you are like most of my patients, you have the following question on your mind: "When should I use heat and when should I use ice?" This is a controversial topic. If you ask ten different doctors or ten different therapists, you may get ten different answers. My opinion has evolved based on research and experience. Here are the basics of where I stand.

Ice makes soft tissues contract and get smaller. Remember the third-grade experiment where you put a balloon filled with air in the freezer to study the effect of cold? When you checked it later, the balloon was smaller. So ice works well to shrink swelling and inflammation in an injured joint.

Heat makes soft tissues expand and get bigger. Think of the flame that is used to fill a hot air balloon. The heat makes the air expand and fill the balloon. So heat helps open up blood vessels to increase circulation and relax muscle spasm.

This is all you have to remember. If you have an injury to a joint, use ice. If you have an injury to a muscle, use heat. Most importantly, *don't overdo it.* Don't use ice or heat longer than ten minutes at a time. There are two reasons for this. First, you can burn or get frostbite. Second, your body will acclimate to the ice or heat and then both therapies lose their beneficial effect and can actually have a detrimental effect.

The past few years have seen renewed controversy regarding ice, which used to be an unquestioned staple of treatment after injury or surgery. In 1978, a physician named Gabe Mirkin wrote a best-selling sports medicine book and coined the term "RICE," which stands for rest, ice, compression, and elevation. Until very recently, RICE was the accepted protocol for the first few days after injury. But in 2014, Dr. Mirkin began to speak out against the use of ice, citing research that showed that ice had either no effect or a detrimental effect.

In 2016 I began to notice that some surgeons instructed their patients not to use ice after surgery. Since then I have taken a harder look at the research, much of which is still contradictory or inconclusive. But a few main findings are clear.

First, ice has been shown to have either no effect or a detrimental effect on muscle injuries.[2,3,4,5,6] Second, ice has been shown to decrease pain and swelling when applied for no more than ten minutes at a time during the first few days after injury.[7] And third, cold compression devices have been shown to have a beneficial effect when used in the first forty-eight hours after knee surgery.[8] I will continue to follow the research, but as of this writing, I recommend ice on joint injuries for no more than ten minutes at a time.

A few other treatments can decrease inflammation. Over-the-counter medications such as ibuprofen and naproxen work well but should be used with caution. The most serious side effect is irritation to the lining of the digestive tract, which can cause bleeding, so if you take blood thinners or have a history of bleeding problems, you should not take these medications. If you are in doubt, check with your doctor. Food can act as a buffer and help prevent irritation, so don't take these medications on an empty stomach.

Other over-the-counter products like Aspercreme and Myoflex contain anti-inflammatory medications, and prescription creams and slow-release patches can have stronger, longer-lasting effects.

If inflammation is severe, your physician may prescribe a stronger anti-inflammatory medication or administer a steroid injection. If this treatment works, your physician may still recommend physical therapy to address the underlying problems. Medications and injections wear off, and if underlying causes are not addressed, inflammation often returns.

A multitude of over-the-counter creams and ointments can relieve or reduce pain even though they do not reduce inflammation. Common brands include Tiger Balm, Salonpas, Thermacare, Bengay, IcyHot, and Biofreeze. Some of these products contain methyl salicylate, which causes a burning sensation that often feels good; it is actually a superficial skin irritant that causes local inflammation, which overtakes the pain of the injury.

Soaking in Epsom salt is another home remedy that has been used for hundreds of years. Epsom salt is actually magnesium sulfate, and it is called a salt because of its chemical composition. Don't put it on your food. Epsom is actually a town in Surrey, England, where the salt was found in natural springs. There is no clinical evidence that supports this treatment, and some researchers believe that the hot water, with or without the salts, is what makes you feel better. But it is safe, and many patients swear by it. And it certainly works better than salad oil.

All of these measures will help keep inflammation, swelling, and muscle spasm under control, but they may not eliminate them altogether. These protective mechanisms can be stubborn. Even if you do everything right, they can come and go for weeks or months. If you have "good and bad days," the protective mechanisms are most likely causing most of your pain. If the injury itself was causing the pain, it would hurt all the time. You wouldn't have "good days." But inflammation, swelling, and muscle spasm can fluctuate. They ebb and flow like a wave. Many things affect them, including your diet, body chemistry, fluid intake, sleep, activity level, mood, and the weather. They are touchy—so touchy in fact that some people have flare-ups with no injury. Sleeping in an awkward position can cause a flare-up. You might get lucky, but be prepared for the possibility that you may have to deal with some recurring inflammation, swelling, or muscle spasm well into the healing process or even after your injury has healed.

RESTORE NORMAL RANGE OF MOTION

Injured soft tissue often contracts and shortens, or becomes tight, resulting in decreased range of motion. This happens for two reasons. The first is inflammation. Inflamed tissues thicken and shorten, and adhesions form between the tissue layers. This causes more friction, wear and tear, and yes, more inflammation. It is a vicious cycle. The tighter they get, the more inflamed they get, and the more inflamed they get, the tighter they get.

The second reason injured areas become tight is that you instinctively move these areas less because they hurt. Lack of motion causes tightness even without injury. If you decided to wear a sling for a couple of weeks for no reason, the muscles, tendons, and ligaments of your shoulder and elbow would shorten and these joints would lose range of motion. This is called adaptive shortening. Tight tissues have less room to move, which means increased friction between tissue layers. Friction causes irritation, and irritation causes inflammation.

So here is the bottom line: If range of motion is limited, it is very difficult, if not impossible, to eliminate inflammation. If you maintain or restore normal range of motion as soon as safely possible, inflammation can subside and healing quality will improve.

RESTORE NORMAL STRENGTH

The muscles around an injured area often become weak. This happens for two reasons. First, the muscles themselves may be injured. Second, as with range of motion, you tend not to move areas that hurt, so the muscles atrophy due to lack of use.

Weak tissues heal weak. Tissues become stronger in response to stress. This is a basic principle of strength training, and it applies to healing tissues as well. If there is no stress on tissues as they heal, they will heal weak or not at all. Now, you need to be careful because some injuries require no stress during the initial phase of healing, because if there is movement between the disrupted structures, healing will not occur. These are called unstable injuries. After unstable injuries have started to heal, stress must be introduced very slowly and gradually. For this reason, it is very important to have a physician evaluate your injury to determine if it is stable or unstable.

This concept applies to bones as well. Bones become weak and brittle in the absence of stress. This is why astronauts must perform resistance training in space. Their healthy bones would become so weak without gravity that they would break under their body weight when they returned to earth. As with soft tissue, stress must be introduced slowly and gradually to healing bones.

RESTORE NORMAL MOVEMENT PATTERNS

Weakness and tightness cause abnormal movements. Limping is a common example, but abnormal movements can occur anywhere. If you watch people with injured shoulders try to reach overhead, they will often hike their shoulders to get their arms up. Abnormal movements cause abnormal forces on joints, and over time can cause more pain, wear and tear, and damage than the original injuries. They can also cause inflammation, swelling, and muscle spasm to persist and impede the healing process.

Abnormal movement patterns can also turn into habits and persist even after you restore full range of motion and strength. Even if you pay attention, you might not realize your movements are abnormal, and correcting them can be the most difficult and complicated part of the process.

PUTTING THEM TOGETHER

Movement is the key to optimal healing. Move too much, and you risk reinjury. Move too little, and you heal tight and weak. Move incorrectly, and you create more wear and tear. The proper amount and type of movement is different for each injury, so it is critically important to learn what is safe and appropriate for your situation.

11

SOLVING MYSTERIES

My first year of physical therapy school was the most intense learning experience of my life. Gross anatomy, neuroanatomy, physiology, kinesiology, biomechanics. Hours upon hours in the cadaver lab. Long, weary nights of studying. Five hours of sleep per night. Coffee.

Then it came time for my first clinical internship. I was finally working with patients, and I couldn't wait for the opportunity to show off the vast stockpile of information that I had downloaded into my brain. This chance came quickly when one of my first patients asked me a question more difficult than anything I had anticipated: "How long before I can ride my bike again?" My first reaction was to say, "Don't you want to know the medical terms for all of the muscles and ligaments that you injured?" But I quickly caught myself, hesitated for only a second, and came right out with, "Uh . . . I'm not really sure; let me go get my instructor."

At that moment I realized that I was not yet a physical therapist and that my real education would consist of many years of practice grappling with tough questions. Questions like, "My husband fell off a stool in our bedroom, and he said that when he hit the hardwood floor, he bounced. Is that possible? Can a person really bounce off the floor?"

This actual question is just one of many that has helped me develop clinical judgment. Clinical judgment is the ability to pretend to take every single question seriously. It is what allows me to say something like, "Absolutely, people bounce like that all the time," without feeling at all guilty about the fact I have no freaking idea if people bounce off hardwood or not.

Today, after twenty-five years of developing clinical judgment, I can answer that question and many others effortlessly. Here are a few real-life examples of exchanges between my patients and me:

Patient (an eighty-seven-year-old man): Can I do somersaults?

Me: Why do you want to do somersaults?

Patient: What exercise can I do to get rid of this sagging flab on the back of my arms?

Me: The Insanity P90XXL Advanced Maniac Edition workout.

Me: Is your pain better or worse now than when you arrived here today?

Patient: I'm not sure; what do you think?

Me: Well, let me see, does it hurt when I do this?

Patient: Aaaaaaacccccccchhhhh!

So as you can see, I have developed the ability to quickly respond to a vast array of complex issues. But to this day, the toughest question of all comes from patients who ask, "Nothing happened, so why does it hurt?" These patients had no injury. They have pain that seemed to come out of nowhere. They woke up with pain, or it started while they were sitting on their recliners watching television, or it came on gradually over several weeks. Whatever the case, they are baffled.

Unexplained pain is actually quite common, and patients who have it are very often frustrated because they have a hard time getting answers. They say, "My doctor doesn't know what's going on," or "The X-rays didn't show anything," or "My last therapist had me doing all this stuff, but I think he was grasping at straws." So what I will do here is take you through my thought process, describe what I tell patients in this situation, and explain why I use certain techniques and methods to deal with unexplained pain. My goal is that after reading this chapter, you will be able to have a productive discussion with your therapist and understand why your therapist is doing certain things in their effort to help you solve the mystery of why you are hurting.

There are several reasons why pain can arise with no traumatic injury. I will discuss the ones that I see most often: defense mechanisms, tightness, weakness, and abnormal movement patterns.

DEFENSE MECHANISMS

As I discussed in chapter 9, defense mechanisms (inflammation, muscle spasm, and scar tissue) are your body's reactions to something. This *something* can be anything from a traumatic injury to a seemingly insignificant event like falling asleep in an awkward position. Once something triggers a defense mechanism, a subsequent chain of events can lead to significant pain and disability. A frozen shoulder is a good example. This condition comes on gradually and progresses to the point where the shoulder is so tight and painful that normal activities become impossible.

If you came to me with a frozen shoulder, you would likely ask me, "Why did this happen?" I would tell you that it probably started with a precipitating event so insignificant that you don't even remember it. You may have lifted something a little too heavy, or reached behind you to grab something out of the back seat of the car, or slept on your arm in an unnatural position. You might have felt a little twinge, but it was probably no worse than a million other little twinges you feel on a typical day. But this twinge happened to trigger inflammation. Over time, this inflammation worsened to the point where it caused pain. Inflammation also causes soft tissues to become thicker and tighter than normal, so your shoulder gradually lost range of motion. You noticed that you couldn't reach as far with that arm. When you tried, it hurt, so you favored the arm and used the other arm most of the time. This lack of use resulted in adaptive shortening (remember this from chapter 9), and the shoulder became even tighter as a result of disuse. The tighter it got, the more inflamed it got, and the more inflamed it got, the tighter it got. You had entered the vicious cycle. On top of all this, your shoulder muscles became weak from disuse, and adhesions (scar tissue) started to form between the tissue layers. So here you are with a shoulder that is weak, tight, inflamed, and painful.

This chain of events can occur anywhere in the body. It is a basic domino effect:

1. Something minor triggers inflammation or muscle spasm (or both).
2. Inflammation and muscle spasm cause pain.
3. Pain leads to disuse.
4. Disuse results in adaptive shortening and atrophy. (You become tight and weak.)
5. Adaptive shortening and atrophy cause abnormal movement.
6. Abnormal movement causes friction and irritation to the moving parts of the joint.
7. Adhesions form, causing more friction and irritation.
8. Friction and irritation lead to more inflammation and muscle spasm.
9. Go to step 2. Repeat.

TIGHTNESS

In the above scenario, tightness is in the middle of the cycle. But tightness can also be the original cause of the problem, resulting in the following cycle:

1. Muscles or ligaments are tight.
2. Tightness causes abnormal movement.
3. Abnormal movement causes friction and irritation to the moving parts of the joint.
4. Adhesions form, causing more friction and irritation.
5. Friction and irritation lead to inflammation and muscle spasm.
6. Inflammation and muscle spasm cause pain.
7. Pain causes disuse.
8. Disuse causes tightness.
9. Go to step 1. Repeat.

This is basically the same cycle with a different starting point. So your next question is, of course, "Why is it tight?" (No, I'm not psychic. I've just heard this question a million times.) The answer is, if I picked a hundred random people off the street, I could probably find tight soft tissues on ninety-nine of them. Those who are genetically gifted, and those who stretch consistently, may have perfect flexibility. But even many people who stretch have areas that are tight. I stretch every day, and I have the flexibility of a coffee table. This is because I am not genetically flexible and I am fifty-six years old. So why do I bother stretching? Because if I didn't, I would be even tighter. I once heard the comedian Will Ferrell joke that he has to run just to stay fat. You work with what you have.

WEAKNESS

Take the above cycle and substitute "weak" for "tight" and you have a vicious cycle that originates with weakness. "Why is it weak?" you ask. The answer is similar, with one slight difference. If I picked a hundred random people off the street, I could find at least one weak muscle on all of them. I have found weak muscles on bodybuilders. Even people who lift weights religiously have weak areas, because they often neglect small, deep muscle groups.

ABNORMAL MOVEMENT PATTERNS

Abnormal movement patterns can also be the root cause of the problem. Just switch the starting point of the cycle. If you don't believe there are random abnormal movement patterns lurking out there, sit on a bench at a mall for an hour and watch people walk around.

Now for your final question: "How do you know which of these four things started the problem?" You don't. And you don't need to worry about it, because it doesn't matter. It's the old question, "Which came first, the chicken or the egg?" Regardless of where it started, you and your therapist still have four main jobs: calm down the defense mechanisms, stretch what is tight, strengthen what is weak, and correct abnormal movement. The goal is not to find the exact cause of your unexplained pain. The goal is to find and correct the mechanical abnormalities. If you do this properly, your pain will most likely resolve.

You may notice that your therapist will look for abnormalities in parts of your body far away from the pain. This is because the body is what we call a closed chain system, which means that every part is connected to every other part. Your arm swing affects the motion of your legs when you walk. Your ankle flexibility affects your stride length, which in turn affects the motion of your low back. If your shoulder is tight, you may have to twist your hips more to reach something. So if you are being treated for low back pain, your therapist may decide to stretch your calf muscles. And if you have been reading carefully, you will not be like all of the other patients who ask, "Why are you stretching my calf muscles when I'm here for my low back?"

When you work to correct abnormal movement patterns, it is especially important to address areas away from the pain. In fact, if you focus too much attention on movement patterns at the painful site, you can sometimes make these movement patterns worse. To understand why, you need to understand some basic physiology of how the nervous system is wired. Many movement patterns are hardwired in the spinal cord, not in the brain. Walking is a good example. You don't have to consciously think about walking; you do it automatically while thinking about many other things. The hardwired program in the spinal cord executes the motion without the brain's help. That is why a chicken with its head cut off can run around. So if you think too much about walking, you can screw up the natural motion of the program your spinal cord is trying to execute. This program is far more complex than the highest-level computer programs ever developed to date by humans. The most sophisticated robots that are programmed to walk like humans really don't walk like humans; they walk like robots trying to walk like humans, and you can easily see the difference. The coordinated sequence of muscle contractions is vastly complex. Your spinal cord is full of hardwired programs that smoothly coordinate movements that you don't even think about. The thinking part of your brain is simply not wired to create such smooth, coordinated movements. So if you think too hard, your movements may be clumsy and awkward.

A simple technique that often works is to focus your attention away from the painful area. For example, if the bottom of your heel hurts when you walk, then think about the motion of your head, or the swing of your arms, or an object at the other side of the room. I found out by accident how well this can work. In the middle of one of my six-month bouts of heel pain, I strained my back helping a patient get onto a treatment table. After about four hours of working through the back pain, I suddenly realized that, for the first time in months, my heel felt fine. I was focused on my back pain, not my foot. The thinking part of my brain got out of the way and allowed my body to do what it automatically knows how to do: walk correctly.

So if your therapist asks you to perform an activity while thinking about something that seems to make no logical sense, have faith. They probably know what they are talking about.

12

PERIPHERAL NEUROPATHY

A Case Study

When I walked Frank Ward back to the exam table on that February day in 2010, I had no idea that, years later, his name would appear in the very first line of my book. Frank not only gave permission, but enthusiastically encouraged me to share his story with as many people as possible, and I do this for several reasons. First, to reveal the awesome power of determination, belief, and persistence: in other words, the power of the *mind*. Second, to demonstrate that physical therapy can have a profound and positive effect on not only injuries but devastating medical conditions. And third, to describe how research is an ongoing process of discovery, not a fixed statement of truth. If you challenge what research suggests, you may open up a whole new path that redefines conventional wisdom.

Peripheral neuropathy causes damage to the nerves of the arms and legs. Symptoms include weakness, numbness and tingling, partial or total paralysis, and constant, severe nerve pain. Causes include traumatic injury, infection, smoking, diabetes, or, in Frank's case, an adverse reaction to medication.

Frank's doctors had told him that physical therapy would not reverse or slow down the progression of his peripheral neuropathy and, as I mentioned on page 1, that he might very well end up in a wheelchair. But Frank was having none of this. He had knee pain from old football injuries, so he convinced one of his doctors to prescribe physical therapy to work on his knees.

Frank described to me his previous experience with physical therapy. His first therapist feared worsening Frank's symptoms and prescribed only basic, easy exercises. Frank asked if he could progress to more difficult exercises. His therapist said no.

Frank saw several other therapists in different clinics and had the same experience with each one. He continued to lose strength, and his ability to walk deteriorated.

Physical therapists must navigate carefully. They walk a fine line between pushing their patients too hard and not pushing hard enough. This delicate balance differs for each patient, and every therapist has their own comfort level with regard to risk-taking. It is easy for therapists to criticize the decisions of previous therapists who have not had good results, and I want to make it clear that I have no issue with Frank's previous therapists following their best clinical judgement. But I do have an issue with the way Frank told me he was treated. His previous clinicians gave him virtually no direction or encouragement. Their attitude toward him was dismissive. They made it clear that his goals were unrealistic, so there was no collaboration. They didn't listen.

In my opinion, Frank had nothing to lose. With the benefit of knowing how Frank had responded to light exercises, I decided that a controlled progression to more aggressive therapy was appropriate. It was not without risk, and the potential benefits were not guaranteed. I discussed this with Frank until we were on the same page. We made a plan and got to work.

Frank attracted a lot of attention in the physical therapy gym. He made a lot of noise. He grunted, groaned, yelled. The aggressive college football player trapped in that broken fifty-five-year-old body fought to get out. If I told him to do twenty repetitions, he would do twenty-five, or thirty, or as many as he could. Frank's determination was contagious, and other patients worked harder when he was around.

Frank gives me all the credit, but I actually did very little. Most of the exercises were his idea. Every day he wanted to try something new, and as time went on I realized that my job was to say, "Sure, let's give it a try," or, "No, I don't think that's a good idea just yet." I very rarely said no.

Three months after we met, Frank walked up and down a flight of fourteen stairs without my help and without holding onto the railing. Frank outweighed me by more than a hundred pounds, and it took some convincing for him to believe that I could safely guard him on the way down and catch him if he stumbled. Lucky for me, my instincts were correct, and he made it without a hitch. He struggled to hold back tears, as did I.

Three months after that he walked up and down the same stairs thirty times without stopping.

Nine months later he was up on his toes and could almost run up and down the flight of stairs. Two weeks after that I started timing him: ten flights in two minutes, twenty-three seconds.

Seven months later, ten flights in two minutes, eight seconds.

Frank often traveled for his job and sought out hotels based on the quality of their gyms and the accessibility of stairwells during all hours. Once, a manager was called to investigate a loud clamor coming from a stairwell at three in the morning. After hearing Frank's story, the manager let him continue. (Being 6-foot-4 and 270 pounds has its advantages.)

Around this time, Frank told me that his doctor said the following: "New research is showing that aggressive, high intensity physical therapy can sometimes reverse the progression of peripheral neuropathy." No kidding.

Frank often made time to talk with other patients who were struggling. He told them his story of how low he had been and how far he had come. He encouraged them, inspired them, and gave them hope.

His effect on me and other therapists was profound. His name always comes up when my colleagues and I reminisce about memorable patients, and I often tell his story to those who believe they will never get better.

I was no magician, and I continue to believe that Frank succeeded because of Frank, not me. But very recently Frank managed to convince me that the things I did were "extremely rare and immensely valuable." These things had nothing to do with intelligence or talent or clinical skill. They were simple: I showed him respect. I gave him a chance. I created an atmosphere of positivity and collaboration. I listened. These things were easy. They should not be extremely rare.

Frank now lives in another state, but he stops in the clinic to see me when he is in town. He is sixty-five and regularly competes in three-mile road races.

PART IV

TREATMENTS FOR INJURIES

13

ALTERNATIVE THERAPIES

At this point many of you are probably thinking, "Boy, this physical therapy thing is a lot of work. You want me to stretch, train for endurance, build strength, change my whole diet around, and somehow still have time to sleep more. Can't I just go somewhere and have someone work on me?" If you are one of these people, you're in luck, because there are other options. I am not an expert on any of them, but I can give you a little information about a few alternative treatments that might be a little easier to fit into your schedule.

REIKI

Reiki is a well-known Japanese healing technique in which practitioners transfer their unseen life force energy to patients through therapeutic touch. Reiki is based on the theory that injury and disease occur when this life force energy is low, so a boost from someone who has a little extra in the tank helps to achieve better healing and health. Over time Reiki came to be known as "laying on of hands," although this phrase is biblical in origin and did not originate with Reiki but was applied to it later. Claims by some Reiki practitioners that they successfully perform this technique over the phone have led to some skepticism. In an effort to get to the bottom of this question, I called several physicians to get their opinions, performed a statistical analysis on the responses, and concluded that the probability that a Reiki practitioner will cure me over the phone is higher than the probability that a single doctor will return my call.

ACUPUNCTURE

Acupuncture is a form of traditional Chinese medicine that is thousands of years old. It is based on the theory that energy flows through all living things in channels called meridians, and that blocked meridians interrupt this energy flow and cause pain and disease. Acupuncture practitioners insert needles into various areas of the body to unblock these meridians and restore normal energy flow. This treatment takes advantage of the well-established medical principle that sticking a million needles into your body makes you forget about any pain that made you go to the doctor in the first place.

ACUPRESSURE

Acupressure is similar to acupuncture, only instead of using needles, practitioners apply direct pressure with their fingers and thumbs to specific areas of the body to open up meridians and restore normal energy flow. This treatment utilizes the equally well-established medical principle that digging the fingers into sensitive pressure points like a playful third grader works almost as well as stabbing you with needles.

REFLEXOLOGY

Reflexology is similar to acupressure, except that practitioners apply pressure to specific areas on the feet that correspond to different parts of the body. This treatment is based on the theory that energy channels flow through the body from top to bottom, so every part of the body is located in a channel that exits through a specific part of the foot. This takes acupressure principles to the next level by taking advantage of the phenomenon that digging the fingers into sensitive feet cures you so thoroughly that you will insist you never have to come back for another treatment ever again.

CHIROPRACTIC

The spine is composed of thirty-three vertebrae that are stacked on top of one another. Joints allow motion between twenty-four of these vertebrae, and sometimes one or more of these joints become locked or jammed together, which prevents motion at those levels. Chiropractic treatment is an invaluable option for people with this condition. "High-velocity low-amplitude thrust" is the technical term for what chiropractors do when they crack the spine and unlock these joints.

Many older patients with brittle bones cannot safely tolerate a high-velocity thrust, so many chiropractors also perform soft tissue work, which is similar to a deep massage. This is also a great treatment option for younger patients who are very tense and fearful of getting their spines cracked.

For those patients who are too tense and fearful of even some soft tissue work, there is another option called light touch chiropractic. Practitioners of this method perform very light, gentle tapping on various areas of the body to release tension and channel energy flow.

And for those patients for whom gentle tapping is just too much to bear, some chiropractors perform energy flow treatments where they don't touch the patients at all. Surprisingly, chiropractors have not yet been able to get these treatments to work over the phone, so patients who are too sensitive to show up in person have to be referred to Reiki practitioners.

COLONIC IRRIGATION

Colonic irrigation is one of the more creative treatments I have encountered. The term "colonic" refers to the colon, which is what gets irrigated during colonic irrigation. To rid the body of toxins, a double-hosed system pumps clean water into the rectum through an "in hose," and waste products out of the rectum through an "out hose."

Surprisingly, colonic irrigation has not yet achieved mainstream acceptance, as there are still many people who insist that they achieve adequate irrigation with an old-fashioned number two.

FELDENKRAIS

The Feldenkrais Method is a system of gentle, specific exercises that correct poor posture and inefficient movement patterns. These exercises reinforce coordinated, comfortable movements that improve brain-body connections and decrease stress and pain. Its founder, Moshe Feldenkrais, was a scientist and engineer in World War II, as well as a judo teacher and soccer player. He developed his method in the mid-twentieth century when he realized that he had one of those really cool names that just had to have some sort of method named after it.

ALEXANDER TECHNIQUE

Frederick Matthias Alexander, a Shakespearean orator, developed this technique in the 1890s to deal with the loss of his own voice. He watched his own performances in the mirror, noticed that he was tensing and contracting certain muscles that pulled him into strained postures, and came up with more efficient movement patterns that miraculously restored his voice. Today, actors and performers use his method to improve the projection of their voices, deal with back and neck pain, and improve overall well-being. What I like most about this technique is that it is even more time consuming than physical therapy, so if you are pressed for time, you might as well just keep reading this book and follow my advice.

MY ADVICE

Despite what my ramblings in this chapter may have led you to believe, I actually recommend some of these and other treatment options to many of my patients. While I believe very strongly in my own profession, I am humble enough to know that what I do is not always the only valid option. None of the above treatments will harm you, and some may work better for you. Balance an open mind with healthy skepticism, and factor in personal experience and comfort. And remember, like physical therapy, these alternative treatments are not substitutes for medical diagnoses, so talk to your physician to rule out any serious underlying conditions.

14

SPECIFIC INJURIES

We have finally arrived at the point where I will discuss how to treat the specific injury that prompted you to buy this book. I would like to congratulate you for suffering through so many pages to find the material you can actually use. And now that we are here, I would also like to tell you how pleased I am that you are feeling so much better and can't even remember what your injury was.

If, on the other hand, you still have your injury and have picked up this book in your doctor's waiting room, you still have about three or four hours to wait, which is plenty of time to finish the remaining chapters.

Human beings love to break things up into sections, and medical practitioners are no different. We see this patient as a foot, that one as a shoulder. Many doctors specialize in particular body parts, and patients are drawn to this. A patient with a knee problem will often choose a particular doctor "because all he does is knees." This way of looking at things can be good and bad, and like most philosophies, it should be recognized and used with balance. A professor once asked our class, "How many oceans are in the world?" She smiled as she watched us mentally count them. As we started to call out answers, she challenged us to picture the earth from outer space, without humans and their organizational schemes. Nearly three-quarters of the earth is covered with one large, unbroken, continuous body of water: one ocean.

This is not to say that it is useless or wrong to recognize differences between parts of this ocean. If you plan to swim off the coast of Norway in the middle of winter, you will certainly pack different equipment than your neighbor who is heading to the Caribbean. The human body is the same, and so the following chapters describe the unique particulars of individual body parts and how to address these differences when rehabilitating injuries. But as you read on, keep in the back of your mind the fact that the entire body is made of various forms of the same stuff. There is really only one ocean.

These chapters also describe sample protocols similar to those that I use to rehabilitate specific injuries. I am hesitant to use the word "protocols," because it connotes cookbook recipes that all people must follow the same way. This is not how physical therapists use protocols. We use them as flexible guidelines that we modify to fit each patient's particular circumstance. If I wanted to give you cookbook recipes, I would not have bothered with all of the chapters up to this point. Protocols only work if you understand why you are performing certain exercises, how the exercises should feel, and when to make adjustments. Ideally, you should use what you learn in these chapters to improve the teamwork between you and your therapist. If you can only afford one or two physical therapy visits, or if your doctor just gave you a sheet of exercises to do at home, you can use this knowledge to understand what to expect, recognize when things aren't going well, and know when to change course and seek another opinion.

I organized these chapters by body parts rather than injuries because there is a great deal of overlap between injuries to the same body part. Take the foot and ankle, for example. The protocols for ankle sprains, plantar fasciitis, and Achilles tendinitis are essentially the same. The differences lie in the severity of the injuries and the specific restrictions that must be adhered to. For example, if you have a grade III sprain of the ligaments on the outside of the ankle, your doctor may instruct you not to stretch the foot to the inside for several weeks, so this alters your protocol. This is why you should not use this book to treat injuries without the guidance of your doctor or therapist.

You can, however, use these protocols to treat everyday aches and pains, which over time can turn into serious conditions if they are not addressed. We all get tighter and weaker as we age, so maintaining good flexibility and strength goes a long way in preventing problems down the line. I treat many severe conditions that could have been avoided if people only knew what to do when they first felt a little twinge. However, if you follow a protocol for a couple of weeks and that little twinge does not go away, see your doctor to rule out something serious.

In keeping with the theme of this book, the protocols I will describe are basic. I will not describe complex exercises that require expensive equipment or hands-on instruction to make sure they are done properly. The only pieces of equipment you may need are simple household items like soup cans or water jugs to be used as weights, and basic stretch resistance bands that many physical therapy clinics provide for free. Your therapist may alter some of the exercises based on your particular situation and will likely instruct you in many more specific exercises that are beyond the scope of this book.

Some of the exercises are performed lying down, so if you have a hard time getting up off the floor, do them on your bed. You do not have to do the exercises all in one session. If you are pressed for time, you can break the sessions up throughout the day. Fit them into your schedule any way you can. It doesn't matter when you do them, just do them.

15

FOOT AND ANKLE INJURIES

If there is one thing I have learned about the foot, it is that it is by far the grossest part of the body. I had no knowledge of this for most of my life because I never thought anything was particularly gross. I learned it from my daughters, who each at very young ages informed me that they would absolutely not be pursuing careers in the medical field or any other field that involved the possibility of an interaction with someone's foot.

It turns out that feet are even grosser than notoriously gross body parts, such as colons and rectums. At least these parts have the decency to conceal themselves under several layers of skin. Most people can make it through a typical day without having to feast their eyes on a rectum. But feet are right out there in the open. And according to my daughters, they don't even have to be gnarled with scaly, scabbed skin, ridged yellow toenails, crusty cracked heels, crooked toes, bunions, blisters, and hairy toe knuckles to be gross. Apparently, young, tan, smooth, perfectly proportioned feet are still the grossest things in the world, which makes foot and ankle injuries ideal for treatment in the privacy of your own home, where these hideous appendages won't horrify innocent members of the general public.

Feet support all of your body weight, so they are made of strong, thick tissue. Imagine how sore your hands would get if you had to walk around on them all day. Even though feet are built tough, this load still commonly triggers inflammation or swelling without any traumatic injury, and swelling tends to persist longer in feet because gravity pulls bodily fluids downward. So with or without a traumatic injury, swelling can be a persistent annoyance. I have treated teenage basketball players for ankle sprains who still experienced occasional swelling even after they had fully healed and were back to playing ball without pain or limitation.

Foot pain also tends to move, and it is common to feel pain in a different place every day. This happens because in response to pain, your body unconsciously makes small adjustments to how you walk. These adjustments often cause pain in another part of the foot. Your body then adjusts again to get around this new pain, which causes the pain to move somewhere else, and so on.

Foot and ankle rehabilitation, with or without traumatic injury, involves achieving the four objectives I described in chapter 10: decrease the body's response, restore normal range of motion, restore normal strength, and restore normal movement patterns. If your doctor or therapist instructed you to follow restrictions, you should alter this protocol so that you do not break those restrictions.

DECREASE THE BODY'S RESPONSE

The first order of business is to decrease inflammation and swelling. Ice and elevation help, but muscle contractions help even more, because they are what prevent your feet and legs from swelling when you are not injured. The veins that carry blood upward and away from your legs contain valves that prevent backflow. When your muscles contract, they squeeze blood up through the veins the same way you squeeze water out of a squirt bottle. The valves prevent this blood from flowing back down to the feet. So among the best exercises to do with any foot or ankle injury are simple ankle pumps. Just pump your ankle up and down as if pushing and releasing a gas pedal. That's it. Many patients do not bother with this exercise because it's so simple that they can't believe it's actually doing anything. Trust me, it is. Just pull your foot back as far as you can, then push it down as far as you can, slow and controlled, about thirty times. In addition to performing this exercise once every hour, apply ice with elevation for ten minutes, two or three times per day, and that is the treatment for inflammation and swelling.

RESTORE NORMAL FLEXIBILITY

Don't wait until the inflammation and swelling have decreased before you work on flexibility. Start right away. In fact, start now, even if you have never had a foot or ankle injury, because doing so may prevent you from ever needing to use this chapter.

The four motions of the ankle are called dorsiflexion (pulling the foot back), plantar flexion (pushing the foot down), inversion (turning the ankle inward), and eversion (turning the ankle outward).

Dorsiflexion is the most important motion, because you need adequate dorsiflexion to achieve a proper, straight ahead push-off during gait. If dorsiflexion is limited, you will unconsciously alter your gait pattern to achieve push-off: You may roll the ankle in, or turn the toe out, or lift the heel up early, or any number of other compensations that cause abnormal stress on various parts of your foot and ankle.

Perform the following exercises twice per day to stretch dorsiflexion.

Towel Calf Stretch

Sit on the floor with your legs straight out in front. Place a towel around the ball of your foot, keep your foot relaxed, keep the knee straight, and pull back on the towel to stretch your foot toward you. Pull the inside of your foot a little harder than the outside to angle your foot inward just a little. Hold the stretch for a count of ten, then relax for a second; repeat this ten times. You should feel a stretch in your calf, back of your ankle, or back of your knee. Stop if you feel pain in the front of your foot, ankle, or knee.

Wall Calf Stretch

Stand facing a wall with your good leg forward and your injured leg back. Keep your back knee straight, your back foot pointing straight ahead or slightly inward, and your back heel on the floor while you lean into the wall. Hold the stretch for a count of ten, then relax for a second; repeat this ten times. You should feel a stretch in your calf, back of your

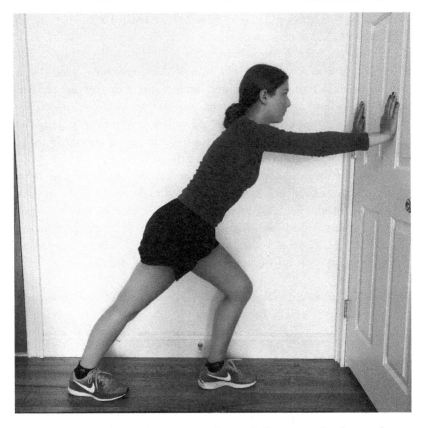

ankle, or back of your knee. Stop if you feel pain in the front of your foot, ankle, or knee.

Restore Normal Strength

The muscles in your foot and ankle have to contract and relax in a smooth, coordinated way, so strength training must incorporate exercises that prompt your muscles to work together and fire at the right times. But first, you should strengthen the four individual motions (dorsiflexion, plantar flexion, inversion, and eversion) separately to ensure that each has enough strength to contribute to the overall system.

Perform the following exercises twice per day to restore strength of these individual movements.

Stretch Band–Resisted Plantar Flexion

Use a stretch band to provide resistance. Push your foot down, then let it back up using a slow, controlled motion. Repeat twenty times.

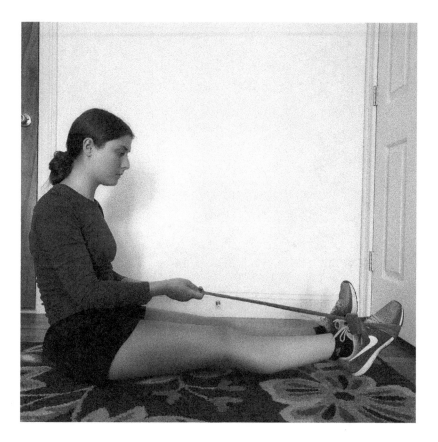

Stretch Band–Resisted Dorsiflexion

Use a stretch band to provide resistance. Pull your foot back, then let it back down using a slow, controlled motion. Repeat twenty times.

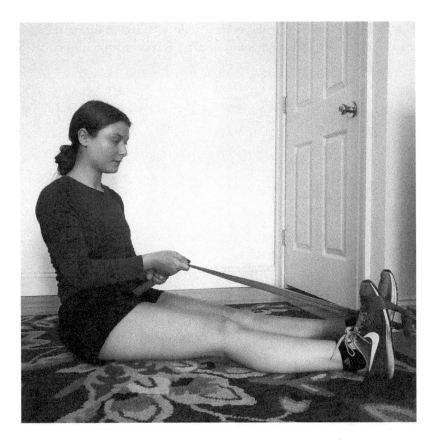

Stretch Band–Resisted Inversion

Use a stretch band to provide resistance. Push your foot inward without rotating your lower leg, then let it back out using a slow, controlled motion. Repeat twenty times.

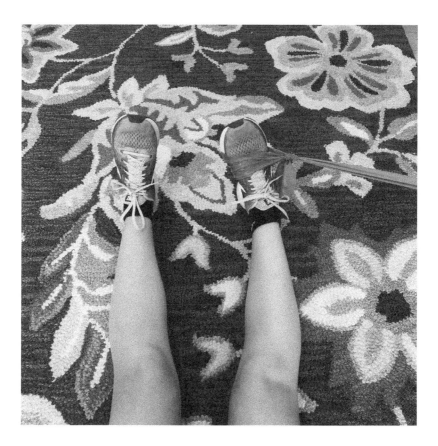

Stretch Band–Resisted Eversion

Use a stretch band to provide resistance. Push your foot outward without rotating your lower leg, then let it back in using a slow, controlled motion. Repeat twenty times.

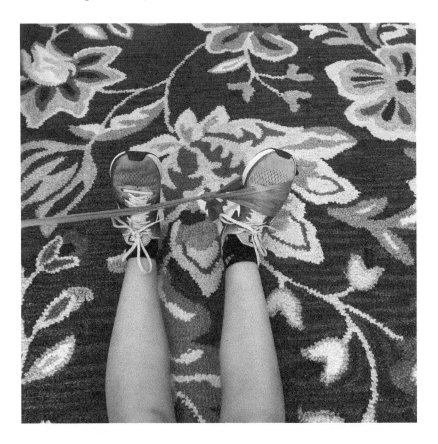

Standing Heel Raise

Stand with your feet shoulder width apart with equal weight on both feet, touch a table or wall for balance, and push up and down on your toes using a slow, controlled motion. Repeat twenty times.

Standing Toe Raise

Stand with your feet shoulder width apart with equal weight on both feet. Hold onto something sturdy like a sink to prevent falling backward, rock back on your heels and lift the balls of your feet up and down using a slow, controlled motion. Repeat twenty times.

RESTORE NORMAL MOVEMENT PATTERNS

The following exercises improve strength as well, but they also force your muscles to work together in a coordinated fashion, or synergy. Improved synergy carries over to everyday activities and helps normalize movement patterns.

Do not try these exercises before you are ready. The exercises should challenge you, but you should not have to struggle to keep your balance. Adequate flexibility and strength of isolated movements are necessary to progress to this stage. Your therapist can help you determine the appropriate time to progress.

Perform the following exercises twice per day to improve movement patterns.

Single-Leg Heel Raise

Stand on your injured leg and push up and down on your toes twenty times using a slow, controlled motion. Touch a table or wall lightly for balance if needed.

Single-Leg Balance

Balance on your injured leg and count to ten, then rest for a few seconds; repeat ten times. Touch a table or wall lightly if needed to keep from falling.

Single-Leg Balance with Leg Swings

Balance on your injured leg and swing your other leg forward and back twenty times, then swing it side to side across the front of your body twenty times. Touch a table or wall lightly if needed to keep from falling.

Heel-to-Toe Walking

Walk heel-to-toe in a straight line for about ten feet, then do it backward to the starting point. Repeat this ten times. Touch a countertop or wall lightly if needed to keep from falling.

16

KNEE INJURIES

Knee injuries are among the most common referrals to physical therapy. Arthroscopic knee surgeries, also known as "knee scopes," have become as routine as dental checkups, and total knee replacements are so common that if you get too close to an orthopedic surgeon, chances are you're getting a new knee, even if you are there for a shoulder problem.

Even our dogs are blowing out their knees. I wish I had a dollar for everyone I know whose dog has had knee surgery. My brother-in-law's dog had two ACL repairs, like he plays for the Packers or something.

So why do we have so many knee injuries? One reason is purely mechanical. The knee moves in only one direction, like a door hinge. The ankle moves up and down, side to side, and rotates. The hip, spine, and shoulder do the same thing. The knee bends in only one plane, and it only goes in one direction in that plane. This is a problem because even those of us who don't make our living playing sports or chasing criminals do a lot of bending, twisting, and side-to-side movements in our daily lives. These activities make it very easy for the knee to move in a direction it is not supposed to go, and when that happens, things get jammed, bruised, torn, and inflamed.

The back of the knee is an area of particular concern with any knee injury, because the soft tissues behind the knee have an exceptional tendency to become inflamed and tight. This can lead to a condition called a knee flexion contracture, which is an inability to fully straighten the knee. A knee flexion contracture can develop quickly after injury or surgery, or it can evolve slowly over many years. A knee that does not fully straighten makes that leg functionally shorter than the other leg, which alters the gait pattern and puts excessive stress on the ankle, hip, and back.

Knee rehabilitation, with or without traumatic injury, involves achieving the four objectives that I described in chapter 10: decrease the body's response, restore normal range of motion, restore normal strength, and restore normal movement patterns. If your doctor or therapist instructed you to follow restrictions, you should alter this protocol so you do not break those restrictions.

DECREASE THE BODY'S RESPONSE

As with the ankle, ice and elevation help decrease inflammation and swelling, but movement and muscle contraction help even more. Inflammation and swelling thrive when there is no movement. Excess fluid pools and sits like water in a pothole. Gentle early motion pumps this fluid out of the joint and prevents the soft tissues from tightening. So once every hour, slowly bend your knee as far as you can, then straighten your knee as far as you can, thirty times. In addition to this, apply ice for ten minutes, two or three times per day, and that is the treatment for inflammation.

RESTORE NORMAL FLEXIBILITY

The two motions of your knee are called flexion (how far the knee bends), and extension (how far the knee straightens). Don't wait until the inflammation and swelling have decreased before you work on flexibility. Start right away, particularly for extension, because you can prevent or reverse a knee flexion contracture if you stretch the soft tissues in the back of your knee *early*. The longer these tissues sit still, the tighter they get, and the harder it is to restore normal motion. An untreated knee flexion contracture can become permanent in as little as a week or two, so do not *wait* to get the knee *straight*!

Knee flexion, on the other hand, will usually continue to improve slowly over time, so it is not necessary to restore full flexion right away. You can stretch gently, and as long as you make steady progress, flexion should continue to improve. However, if progress halts, you may need more aggressive stretching, which should be done only under the supervision of a physical therapist. In severe cases, flexion may not improve even with aggressive stretching, and you may need a *manipulation under anesthesia*. During this procedure, you are taken to the operating room and placed under general anesthesia. The surgeon then bends your knee slowly but forcefully past the point of limitation to break up scar tissue, and the sound of this scar tissue tearing is often audible. It is the ultimate stretch that you could not tolerate when awake. Do not be afraid of this procedure if you need it. You may be a little sore the next day, but most patients report a significant decrease in pain because their knees finally move freely.

In addition to the knee itself, you should also stretch the muscles that cross the knee. The calf and hamstring both cross the back of the knee, so stretching these muscles helps improve knee extension. The quadricep crosses the front of the knee, so stretching this muscle helps improve knee flexion.

Perform the following exercises twice per day to improve knee extension.

Quad Set

Sit on the floor with your legs straight. Contract your thigh muscle to push your knee as straight as possible. Hold this contraction and count to ten, then relax for a second; repeat ten times.

Passive Knee Extension Stretch

Sit on the floor with your legs straight. Keep your leg relaxed and push your knee straight with your hands. Hold and count to ten, then relax for a second; repeat ten times.

Prone Hang

Lie on your stomach on a bed with your lower leg and knee hanging off the edge. Keep your leg relaxed and let it hang straight for five minutes. Stop early if pain becomes severe.

Hamstring Stretch

Lie on your back, place a towel around your foot, keep your leg relaxed, and pull on the towel to stretch your leg up toward the ceiling. Keep your knee straight or slightly bent. Keep your other leg straight. Hold the stretch for a count of ten, then relax for a second; repeat this ten times. You should feel a stretch in the back of your thigh or knee. Stop if you feel pain in the front of your hip or knee.

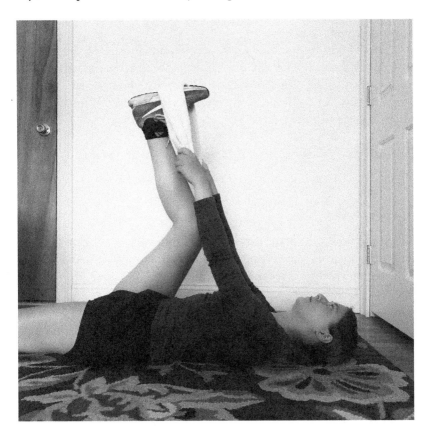

Towel Calf Stretch

Sit on the floor with your legs straight out in front. Place a towel around the ball of your foot, keep your foot relaxed, keep the knee straight, and pull back on the towel to stretch your foot toward you. Pull the inside of your foot a little harder than the outside to angle your foot inward just a little. Hold the stretch for a count of ten, then relax for a second; repeat this ten times. You should feel a stretch in your calf, back of your ankle, or back of your knee. Stop if you feel pain in the front of your foot, ankle, or knee.

Wall Calf Stretch

Stand facing a wall with your uninjured leg forward and your injured leg back. Keep your back knee straight, your back foot pointing straight ahead or slightly inward, and your back heel on the floor while you lean into the wall. Hold the stretch for a count of ten, then relax for a second; repeat this ten times. You should feel a stretch in your calf, back of your ankle, or back of your knee. Stop if you feel pain in the front of your foot, ankle, or knee.

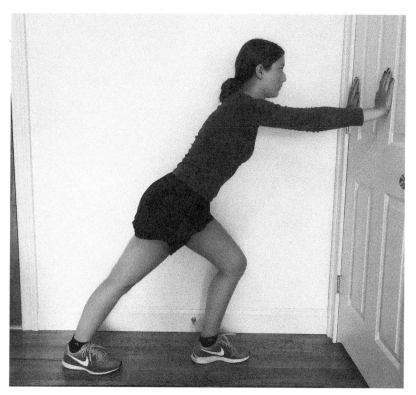

Perform the following exercises twice per day to improve knee flexion.

Heel Slide

Sit on the floor with your legs straight out in front. Place a towel around your foot. Pull on the towel to slide your foot toward you and bend your knee as far as possible. Hold the stretch and count to ten, then slide your foot back down; repeat this ten times. Stop if you feel pain in the back of the knee.

Quad/Hip Flexor Stretch

Lie face up at the edge of a bed and let your injured leg hang off the side. Keep your other knee bent. Place a towel around your foot and

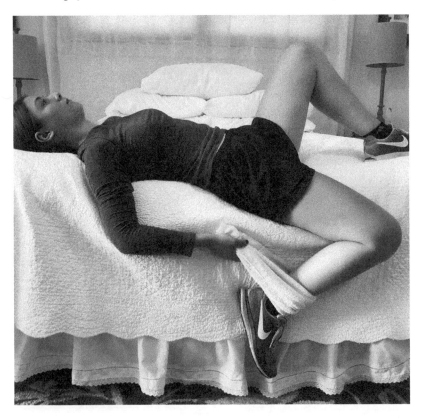

pull on the towel to bend your knee. You should feel a stretch in the front of your knee, thigh, or hip. Stop if you feel pain in your low back or back of your knee.

RESTORE NORMAL STRENGTH

The muscles that surround your knee have to contract and relax in a smooth, coordinated way, so strength training must incorporate exercises that prompt your muscles to work together and fire at the right times. But first, you should strengthen the individual motions (flexion and extension) separately to ensure that each has enough strength to contribute to the overall system.

Most of the muscles of your knee are two-joint muscles, which means that they control either your knee and ankle or your knee and hip. So if your knee is weak, there is a very good chance that your ankle and hip are weak as well. In addition, activities that involve your knee (i.e., walking, running, squatting, etc.) also involve your ankle and hip, so to restore full knee strength, you must also restore full ankle and hip strength.

Perform the following exercises twice per day to restore strength of the individual movements of your knee, ankle, and hip.

Straight Leg Raise

Lie on your back with your injured leg straight and your other leg bent. Tighten your thigh to keep your injured knee as straight as possible, raise your injured leg up to the height of your other knee, then lower your leg; repeat twenty times using a slow, controlled motion.

Side-Lying Hip Abduction

Lie on your side with your injured leg up. Keep your injured knee straight and raise your leg straight up to the side, then lower your leg; repeat twenty times using a slow, controlled motion. Keep your top foot horizontal (don't turn your toes up) and keep your hips square (don't roll your hips back).

Prone Hip Extension

Lie on your stomach. Keep your injured knee straight and raise your injured leg up, then lower your leg; repeat twenty times using a slow, controlled motion. Stop if this causes low back pain.

Adductor Squeeze

Lie on your back with both knees bent and place a pillow between your knees. Squeeze the pillow with both legs, hold this contraction and count to ten, then relax for a second; repeat ten times.

Seated Knee Extension

Sit on a chair. Straighten your injured knee all the way, then bend it back down; repeat twenty times using a slow, controlled motion.

Standing Knee Flexion

Stand and hold a table or countertop for balance. Bend your injured knee as far as you can comfortably by raising your leg, then let it back down; repeat twenty times using a slow, controlled motion.

Standing Heel Raise

Stand with your feet shoulder width apart with equal weight on both feet, touch a table or wall for balance, and push up and down on your toes using a slow, controlled motion. Repeat twenty times.

RESTORE NORMAL MOVEMENT PATTERNS

The following exercises improve strength as well, but they also force your muscles to work together in a coordinated fashion, or synergy. Improved synergy carries over to everyday activities and helps normalize movement patterns.

Do not try these exercises before you are ready. The exercises should challenge you, but you should not have to struggle to keep your balance. Adequate flexibility and strength of isolated movements are necessary to progress to this stage. Your therapist can help you determine the appropriate time to progress.

Perform the following exercises twice per day to improve movement patterns.

Mini-Squat

Stand with your feet shoulder width apart. Rest your hands on a table or countertop for balance. Keep your back straight, squat down partway, then return to standing; repeat twenty times using a slow, controlled motion. Stop if you feel pain in the front of your knee.

Short Lunge

Stand with your feet shoulder width apart. Keep your back straight and step forward with your injured leg to the position shown. Push back to

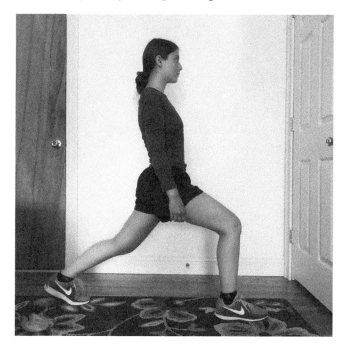

the starting position and repeat with your other leg. Continue to alternate legs and complete ten on each leg. Stop or shorten your step if you feel pain in the front of your knee.

Standing Hip Abduction

Stand and rest your hands on a table or countertop for balance. Raise your injured leg to the side, then let it back down; repeat twenty times using a slow, controlled motion. Repeat with your other leg. Keep your foot pointing straight ahead and don't raise your leg too high. When this becomes easy, tie a stretch band around your ankles to provide resistance.

Standing Hip Extension

Stand and rest your hands on a table or countertop for balance. Raise your injured leg back with your knee straight, then let it back down; repeat twenty times using a slow, controlled motion. Repeat with your other leg. When this becomes easy, tie a stretch band around your ankles to provide resistance.

Side Step

Stand with your knees slightly bent and sidestep across the room for twenty steps, then back the other way for twenty steps. Keep your feet pointing straight ahead. When this becomes easy, tie a stretch band around your ankles to provide resistance.

Single-Leg Heel Raise

Stand on your injured leg and push up and down on your toes twenty times using a slow, controlled motion. Touch a table or wall lightly for balance if needed.

Single-Leg Balance

Balance on your injured leg and count to ten, then rest for a few seconds; repeat ten times. Touch a table or wall lightly if needed to keep from falling.

Single-Leg Balance with Leg Swings

Balance on your injured leg and swing your other leg forward and back twenty times, then swing it side to side across the front of your body twenty times. Touch a table or wall lightly if needed to keep from falling.

17

HIP INJURIES

When I was a student intern at a hospital, I walked into the physical therapy gym where patients who recently had total hip replacements performed exercises. One gentleman was puffing out his cheeks, the way little kids do when they hold their breath. In fact, he looked like he was holding his breath. His face was red and he looked to be on the verge of losing consciousness. I asked him what he was doing. He said his therapist had told him to clench his cheeks together. He hadn't realized that his therapist was talking about his butt cheeks.

This close call could have ended in catastrophe, and as I corrected his technique I was struck by the extraordinary responsibility therapists have to make sure their patients perform exercises correctly. This is especially important when dealing with something as critical as firing your glutes, which, as I mentioned in chapter 5, is an integral component of proper hip function. "Glute" is actually short for "gluteus maximus," which is the technical term for your butt muscle. Actually, your butt comprises several different muscles, so a more accurate definition of the gluteus maximus would be "the largest muscle of your butt." But this description can be deceiving, as some people have extremely prominent glutes, while others appear to have none at all. My uncle's butt is as flat as a touchscreen, and he often jokes that he left his ass in his other pants.

But enough about my uncle's ass. One of the most important things to remember about hip function is that improper movement patterns often cause chronic problems. These can happen anywhere in the body, but they are particularly common with hips. The above-mentioned gluteus maximus, as well as the gluteus medius (a smaller muscle on the side of the hip) are commonly underfired muscles. Improper firing patterns can result from injuries and perpetuate problems, but more importantly, they can occur for no reason and cause damage so slowly that no symptoms are apparent for years. A surprisingly high percentage of people with no history of hip pain or injury have labral tears—and not just older folks. Studies have revealed labral tears in up to a third of people in their twenties and two-thirds of people in their thirties.[1,2,3] Based on what I have observed over the years, I suspect these are at least in part due to improper movement patterns, although research has not yet demonstrated this correlation.

Another unique quality of hip injuries is that they are often mistaken for low back injuries, and vice versa. Many years ago I treated my mother for low back pain for several months before taking her to see a spine specialist, who took an X-ray and found that she needed a hip replacement. Several years later I treated my father for low back pain; he later had an X-ray and found out that he, too, needed a hip replacement. So I'm a little slow, but I do catch on eventually. (This book is way cheaper than your copay.) The hip and the back are connected by many structures, so the injuries often overlap, and many times both areas are involved.

Hip rehabilitation, with or without traumatic injury, involves achieving the four objectives that I described in chapter 10: decrease the body's response, restore normal range of motion, restore normal strength, and restore normal movement patterns. If your doctor or therapist instructed you to follow restrictions, you should alter this protocol so you do not break those restrictions.

DECREASE THE BODY'S RESPONSE

The hip is a deep joint that is located several inches below skin level, so ice will do little for inflammation in the joint itself. But inflammation often occurs in the tendons and bursa, which are closer to the surface, so if this is the case, ice is beneficial. There is no way to know for sure where the inflammation is, but I recommend ice because it can't hurt, and if the inflammation is close to the surface it may help. As with all other joints, gentle motion is the best way to decrease inflammation and swelling. So once every hour, stand next to a countertop, rest one hand on the countertop for balance, keep the knee straight, and gently swing your injured leg forward and backward like a pendulum twenty times. In addition to this, apply ice for ten minutes, two or three times per day, and that is the treatment for inflammation.

RESTORE NORMAL FLEXIBILITY

The hip is a ball-and-socket joint, so it has many planes of motion. It moves forward and back (flexion and extension) and outside and inside (abduction and adduction), rotates to turn the toes in (internal rotation), and rotates to turn the toes out (external rotation).

The hip has a small ball and a deep socket, which makes it stable but not terribly flexible. (Keep this in mind later in chapter 20, where I describe how the shoulder is the exact opposite.) Good stability makes it very difficult to dislocate your hip, but it also makes it difficult to kick over your head. People like gymnasts and contortionists can do this, but average people cannot. The good news is that, for most people, kicking over the head is not a necessary skill, and normal walking, or even slow running, does not require excessive hip motion.

The two basic motions required to walk are flexion and extension. Most injured or inflamed hips become tight in the front, which limits hip extension and causes pain in the front or side of the hip during the push-off phase of gait. This pain often causes the low back to compensate with excessive rotation, and before long the hip injury gives rise to a back injury.

As with all other joints, it is important to stretch the muscles that cross the hip. The hamstring crosses the back of the hip, so stretching this muscle helps improve hip flexion and decrease tension on your back when you swing your leg forward to walk. The hip flexor crosses the front of the hip, so stretching this muscle helps improve hip extension.

Perform the following exercises twice per day to improve hip extension.

Half-Kneeling Hip Flexor Stretch

Kneel on your painful side with your other leg in front with the knee bent and foot flat on the floor. Keep your back straight and glide your hips forward. Hold the stretch and count to ten, then return to the start position for a second; repeat this ten times. You should feel a stretch in the front of your hip and thigh.

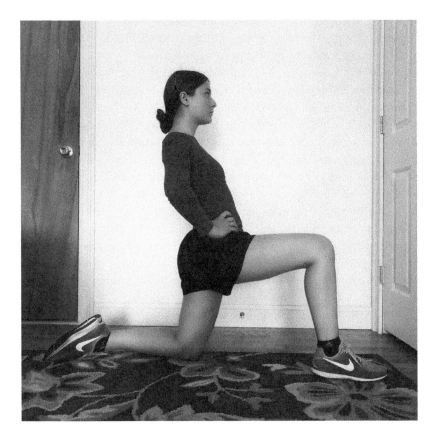

Quad/Hip Flexor Stretch

Lie face up at the edge of a bed and let your injured leg hang off the side. Keep your other knee bent. Place a towel around your foot and pull on the towel to bend your knee. You should feel a stretch in the front of your knee, thigh, or hip. Stop if you feel pain in your low back or back of your knee.

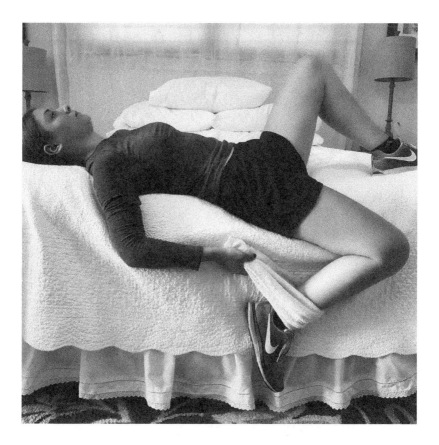

Perform the following exercise twice per day to improve hip flexion.

Hamstring Stretch

Lie on your back, place a towel around your foot, keep your leg relaxed, and pull on the towel to stretch your leg up toward the ceiling. Keep your knee straight or slightly bent. Keep your other leg straight. Hold the stretch for a count of ten, then relax for a second; repeat this ten times. You should feel a stretch in the back of your thigh or knee. Stop if you feel pain in the front of your hip or knee.

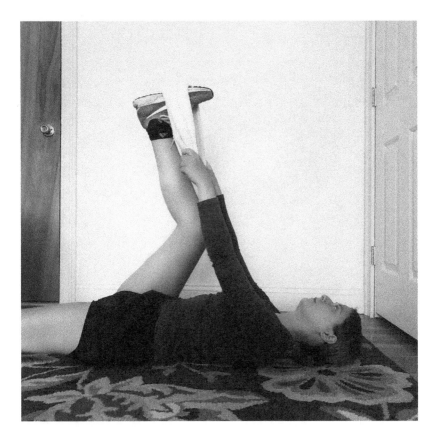

RESTORE NORMAL STRENGTH

The muscles that surround your hip have to contract and relax in a smooth, coordinated way, so strength training must incorporate exercises that prompt your muscles to work together and fire at the right times. But first, you should strengthen the individual motions separately to ensure that each has enough strength to contribute to the overall system. In addition to the above motions of flexion and extension, you should also strengthen abduction and adduction to provide stability around the entire joint.

You may experience a bit of déjà vu while reading this section. Because of the overlap of two-joint muscles between the hip and the knee, some of the exercises to strengthen individual hip motions are also described in chapter 16 to strengthen individual knee motions.

Straight Leg Raise

Lie on your back with your injured leg straight and your other leg bent. Tighten your thigh to keep your injured knee as straight as possible, raise your injured leg up to the height of your other knee, then lower your leg; repeat twenty times using a slow, controlled motion.

Side-Lying Hip Abduction

Lie on your side with your injured leg up. Keep your injured knee straight and raise your leg straight up to the side, then lower your leg; repeat twenty times using a slow, controlled motion. Keep your top foot horizontal (don't turn your toes up) and keep your hips square (don't roll your hips back).

Prone Hip Extension

Lie on your stomach. Keep your injured knee straight and raise your injured leg up, then lower your leg; repeat twenty times using a slow, controlled motion. Stop if this causes low back pain.

Adductor Squeeze

Lie on your back with both knees bent and place a pillow between your knees. Squeeze the pillow with both legs, hold this contraction and count to ten, then relax for a second; repeat ten times.

Bridge

Lie on your back with your knees bent. Tighten your buttock muscles and raise your hips off the floor, then lower your hips back down; repeat twenty times using a slow, controlled motion. Stop if this causes low back pain.

RESTORE NORMAL MOVEMENT PATTERNS

The following exercises improve strength as well, but they also force your muscles to work together in a coordinated fashion, or synergy. Improved synergy carries over to everyday activities and helps normalize movement patterns.

Do not try these exercises before you are ready. The exercises should challenge you, but you should not have to struggle to keep your balance. Adequate flexibility and strength of isolated movements are necessary to progress to this stage. Your therapist can help you determine the appropriate time to progress.

Because of the overlap of two-joint-muscles between the hip and the knee, you will recognize the following exercises from chapter 16.

Perform the following exercises twice per day to improve movement patterns.

Standing Hip Abduction

Stand and rest your hands on a table or countertop for balance. Raise your injured leg to the side, then let it back down; repeat twenty times using a slow, controlled motion. Repeat with your other leg. Keep your foot pointing straight ahead and don't raise your leg too high. When this becomes easy, tie a stretch band around your ankles to provide resistance.

Standing Hip Extension

Stand and rest your hands on a table or countertop for balance. Raise your injured leg back with your knee straight, then let it back down; repeat twenty times using a slow, controlled motion. Repeat with your other leg. When this becomes easy, tie a stretch band around your ankles to provide resistance.

Side Step

Stand with your knees slightly bent and sidestep across the room for twenty steps, then back the other way for twenty steps. Keep your feet pointing straight ahead. When this becomes easy, tie a stretch band around your ankles to provide resistance.

Mini-Squat

Stand with your feet shoulder width apart. Rest your hands on a table or countertop for balance. Keep your back straight, squat down partway, then return to standing; repeat twenty times using a slow, controlled motion.

Short Lunge

Stand with your feet shoulder width apart. Keep your back straight and step forward with your injured leg to the position shown. Push back to the starting position and repeat with your other leg. Continue to alternate legs and complete ten on each leg using a slow, controlled motion.

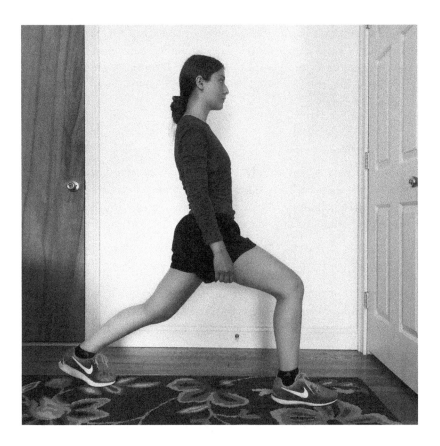

Single-Leg Balance

Balance on your injured leg and count to ten, then rest for a few seconds; repeat ten times. Touch a table or wall lightly if needed to keep from falling.

Single-Leg Balance with Leg Swings

Balance on your injured leg and swing your other leg forward and back twenty times, then swing it side to side across the front of your body twenty times. Touch a table or wall lightly if needed to keep from falling.

18

LOW BACK INJURIES

No body part has done more for the proliferation of therapeutic devices and gadgets than the low back. My favorites over the years have been the ones that allow people to hang upside down like bats. These were born out of the scientifically proven fact that bats do not get low back pain. The first of these, called gravity boots, looked like ski boots with hooks on them that were used to suspend people from rods mounted across doorways. These devices were instrumental in improving the quality of people's lives, especially those who happened to be personal injury lawyers for clients who set the bars up wrong and fell on their heads.

As time went on, researchers found that hanging upside down worked much better when people did not fall on their heads, so safer devices called inversion tables hit the market. A typical inversion table is easy to assemble and comes with a book of warnings that is similar to the operations manual for the space shuttle, only longer.

I use an inversion table with many patients, and I recommend it as a safe way to provide traction to the spine. So imagine my surprise when I recently found out that hanging upside down for too long can result in death.[1] The only thing that surprised me more was that the book of warnings that came with our inversion table did not mention that you could die from hanging upside down for too long. I know there was only so much space, and there were many very helpful safety warnings, like, "Don't hang in the inversion table before you put it together." I mean, I know they couldn't possibly mention *everything*, but it would probably have been a good idea to mention that *you could die from hanging upside down for too long.*

So I instruct patients to limit their time to ten minutes or less. Most people don't even like to hang that long, because after about three or four minutes their ankles get sore. That is plenty of time for traction to have beneficial effects. Don't sleep on your inversion table unless you want your family members to have to deal with your skeletal remains the next morning.

I also don't recommend hanging upside down right after a big meal. Apparently, there was not room for this in the encyclopedia of warnings, either. And of course, if you become dizzy, lightheaded, nauseous, or have increased pain, stop using the inversion table. Traction should feel good. In fact, most research studies actually suggest that the *only* benefit of traction is that it feels good and that for most people it does not affect speed or quality of recovery. However, these same studies suggest that traction *may* improve speed and quality of recovery for *some* people, and you may be one of these people.[2]

Even if you benefit from traction, it should not be your only treatment because it does nothing to correct strength and flexibility deficits. The same four objectives described in previous chapters—decrease the body's response, restore normal range of motion, restore normal strength, and restore normal movement patterns—apply to low back injuries as well, and restrictions imposed by your physician must be followed. But it is important to understand that if your doctor does impose specific restrictions, it is usually because of bony abnormalities or fractures. Restrictions based on soft tissue abnormalities, such as herniated discs, are usually determined by your therapist and are based on your symptoms rather than MRI images, because there is a very low correlation between MRI results and symptoms that require treatment. MRI studies on large numbers of people who had never had symptoms revealed that about half of these people had herniated discs.[3] This means that if you have never had back pain, there is a fifty-fifty chance that you have a herniated disc and don't even know it. It also means that if you do have a back injury and an MRI shows a herniated disc, there is a good chance that the herniated disc has nothing to do with your pain. A test like this is only one piece of the puzzle. A doctor once described it to me this way: An MRI is like a picture of a telephone; you can tell from the picture that it is a telephone, but you can't tell if it is ringing.

Low back injuries can also cause symptoms in one or both legs. All of the nerves in your legs branch off the spinal cord at the low back, and any increase in pressure or tension on these nerves can cause a variety of symptoms such as numbness, tingling, hot or cold sensations, or pain (also known as sciatica) to travel down your leg or arise at a specific part of your hip, leg, or foot. These are called radicular symptoms and can sometimes occur with no back pain at all. When rehabilitating this type of injury, it is important to work closely with your therapist and communicate what you feel during various movements, because this will determine which exercises you will perform. With few exceptions, you should not perform exercises that cause radicular symptoms to increase.

DECREASE THE BODY'S RESPONSE

In the joints of the arms and legs, the body's most pronounced responses to injuries are inflammation and swelling. With back injuries, inflammation and swelling can still occur, but the body's most pronounced response is most often muscle spasm. Back muscles are postural muscles, and the nervous system is wired to cause these muscles to contract automatically, without conscious thought. Muscle spasm, which is an automatic response, kicks in with more vigor in this system that is already wired for automatic contractions.

With other joints, gentle early motion is the best way to decrease the body's response. However, in the first few minutes after a back injury, I have learned from my own experience that the opposite is true. Physical therapists often treat each other, and I've seen therapists strain their backs and immediately launch into stretching and moving and getting other therapists to manipulate their spines and stretch their legs and perform manual techniques. It's like they're going into battle. I have done this myself and have found that, for me, *it doesn't work.* My theory—and this is not based on evidence or research; it is only my theory—is that too much motion in the first few minutes after a back strain tricks my body into thinking that I am injuring myself more, and this causes the muscle spasm to get stronger.

I have found that the best thing to do immediately when I strain my back is to stop moving. I don't even change positions, I just stay where I am. I take slow, deep breaths and focus on relaxing every muscle in my body, especially my back muscles. Then I slowly try to move into a normal standing position while I continue to persuade my entire body to ease and relax. If I can't do this without severe pain, I don't force it. I just stay in the position that is least painful: deep breaths, relax. When I can make it to a chair to sit or to a bed to lie down comfortably, then I do this and continue to breathe and relax as much as possible. In five or ten minutes I am usually able to move a little more easily, but I move slowly. I get up and walk around. I think of it as working with my body, not fighting it. I think of the muscle spasm as a wild animal, like a bear that I stumbled upon in the woods. I imagine moving away as slowly and calmly as possible so I do not startle the bear.

To my knowledge, this technique has never been studied or published, but I have used it several times successfully. I have also described it to patients who have later reported that they too used it successfully. In my opinion, it is your best chance to eliminate muscle spasm quickly. If this technique works for you, I recommend waiting a day before you work on flexibility and strength. This will decrease the chance that the muscle spasm will come fighting back.

Ice and heat can also help decrease the body's response. There may be inflammation, but the joints that are inflamed are deep and covered by several inches of soft tissue, so ice or heat will not penetrate to that level. In my experience, most patients respond well to heat, which helps relax the muscles that are in spasm. Having said that, there are some people who feel worse with heat and better with ice. If you are one of these people, use ice. Remember, neither one does anything to heal your injury, they just make you feel a little better so that you can tolerate the thing that does help you heal—movement.

RESTORE NORMAL FLEXIBILITY

Your low back, or lumbar spine, moves in four directions: flexion (forward bend), extension (backward bend), lateral flexion (side bend), and rotation (twist).

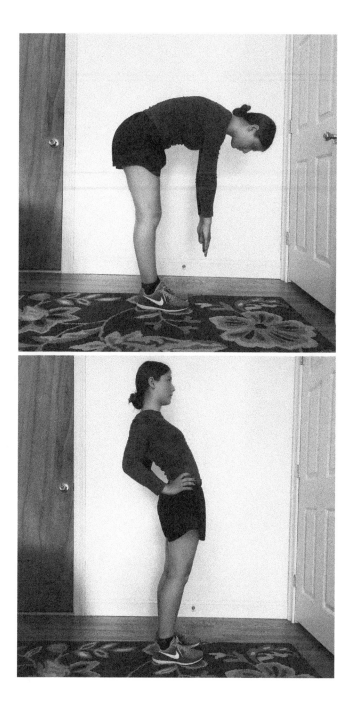

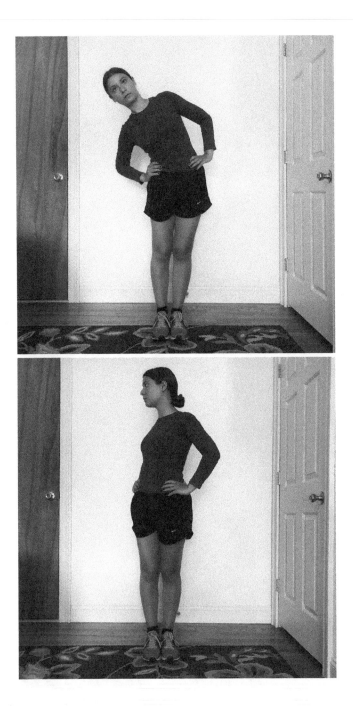

The safest way to use your spine is to minimize these motions. That is, when you lift and move things, especially heavy things, most of the motion should come from your legs. You should hold your back relatively still. Most injuries occur when a spine loaded with heavy weight bends or twists too far, and many people do this because their legs are not flexible.

Even when you are not bending or lifting, tight leg muscles can cause undue stress on your low back because these muscles attach to your pelvis, and your pelvis attaches to your spine. Everything is connected. Tight leg muscles pull too hard on your pelvis, which in turn pulls too hard on your spine. This can create a constant back ache and predispose your spine to injury.

The three most important muscles to stretch are your hamstrings (back of your thigh), quadriceps and hip flexors (front of your thigh and hip), and piriformis. You may not even know that you have a piriformis, but this small muscle can contribute to significant back pain or radicular symptoms.

The piriformis is a deep hip muscle. If you push right in the middle of your buttock, you are pushing on your piriformis. When it contracts, it rotates your hip outward, so if you stand and turn your toes out, you are contracting your piriformis.

The sciatic nerve runs right next to the piriformis, and in about 10 percent of people it goes right through the piriformis, so a tight piriformis can squeeze the sciatic nerve and cause radicular symptoms.

Perform the following exercises twice per day to improve hip and lower extremity flexibility.

Half-Kneeling Hip Flexor Stretch

Kneel on the side to be stretched with your other leg in front with the knee bent and foot flat on the floor. Keep your back straight and glide your hips forward. Hold the stretch and count to ten, then return to the start position for a second; repeat this ten times. You should feel a stretch in the front of your hip and thigh. Repeat on the other side.

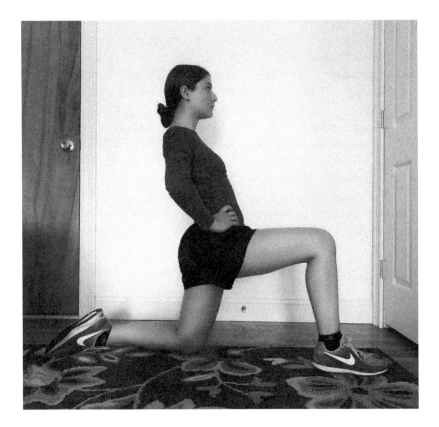

Quad/Hip Flexor Stretch

Lie face up at the edge of a bed and let one leg hang off the side. Keep your other knee bent. Place a towel around your foot and pull on the towel to bend your knee. You should feel a stretch in the front of your knee, thigh, or hip. Stop if you feel pain in your low back or if radicular symptoms become worse. Repeat on the other side.

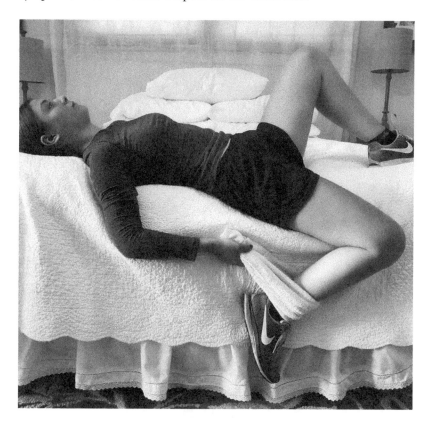

Piriformis Stretch

To stretch the right piriformis, lie on your back and flex your right knee and hip. Hold your right knee with your right hand and your right ankle with your left hand, then pull both diagonally to the left. Hold the stretch and count to ten, then return to the start position for a second; repeat this ten times. You should feel a stretch in the middle of your right buttock. Stop if you feel pain in your groin or front of your hip. Repeat on the other side.

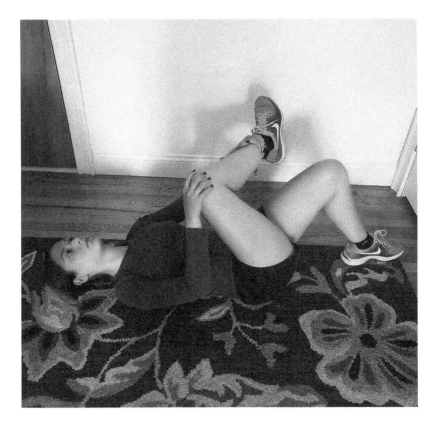

Hamstring Stretch

Lie on your back, place a towel around your foot, keep your leg relaxed, and pull on the belt to stretch your leg up toward the ceiling. Keep your knee straight or slightly bent. Keep your other leg straight. Hold the stretch for a count of ten, then relax for a second; repeat this ten times. You should feel a stretch in the back of your thigh or knee. Stop if you feel increased radicular symptoms or pain in the front of your hip or knee. Repeat on the other side.

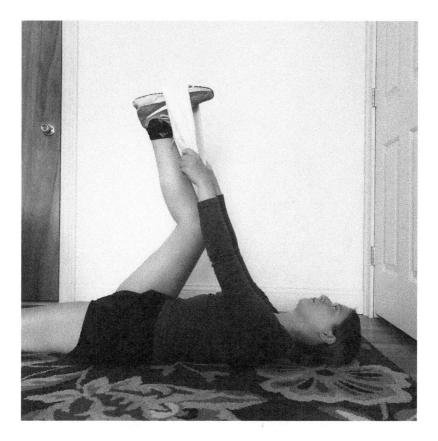

Sciatic Nerve Glide

If the hamstring stretch causes radicular symptoms—nerve pain, numbness, or tingling down the leg—perform the sciatic nerve glide instead. Sit slumped with your head down and arms behind you. Dorsiflex your ankle by pulling your toes up toward you. Hold your ankle in that position and straighten your knee, then immediately bend your knee back down. Do not hold the stretch. Repeat this twenty times on each side using a slow, controlled motion. This is one of the few exercises that is appropriate to perform if it causes increased radicular symptoms during the exercise. If these symptoms persist for more than five minutes after the exercise is complete, then do not perform the exercise again.

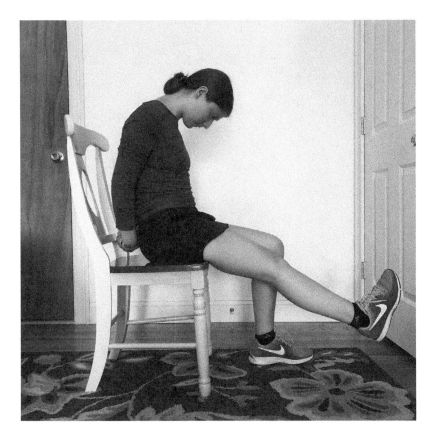

Cat and Camel

Gentle range of motion for lumbar flexion, extension, and rotation helps restore normal motion and decrease inflammation and muscle spasm. The safest way to stretch flexion and extension is on all fours, because in this position your spine does not bear any weight. To improve lumbar flexion and extension, perform the following exercise twice per day.

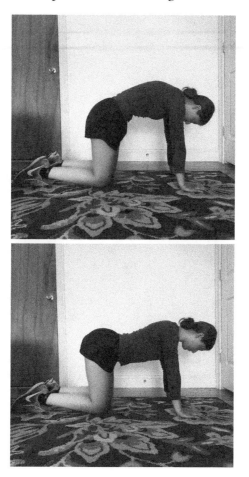

On all fours, round your back up toward the ceiling, hold for a count of three, then arch your back down toward the floor, hold for a count of three. Repeat this twenty times using a slow, controlled motion.

Lower Trunk Rotation

The safest way to stretch rotation is lying on your back, because in this position your spine does not bear any weight. Perform the following exercise twice per day to improve lumbar rotation.

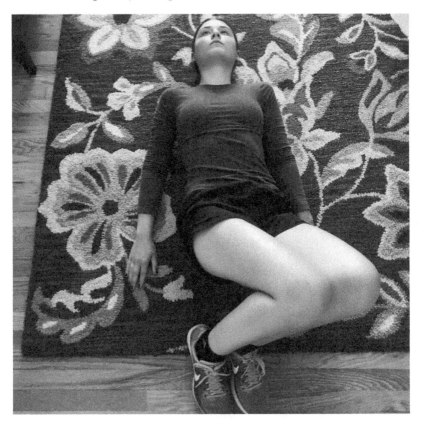

Lie on your back with your knees bent, feet and knees together. Rotate both knees to the right about halfway to the floor, then to the left; repeat twenty times using a slow, controlled motion. Stop or shorten the motion if you have increased pain or radicular symptoms.

RESTORE NORMAL STRENGTH

The most important muscles to strengthen are collectively known as the "core." Your core consists of the muscles of your low back, sides, stomach, hips, and buttocks. When these muscles are strong, they absorb your body weight. When they are weak, more of your body weight goes to the spine. This increases the compressive load on the spine and impedes injuries from healing.

As with muscles that control other joints, the core muscles have to contract and relax in a smooth, coordinated way. But on a more basic level, they have to contract, period. I make this point because I have treated many patients who have adequate core strength but don't contract these muscles during activity. Surprisingly, many of these patients are young, healthy athletes.

Before you incorporate exercises that prompt your muscles to work together and fire at the right times, you should first strengthen the core muscles separately, for two reasons: to ensure that each has enough strength to contribute to the overall system and to teach your nervous system what it feels like to contract each core muscle.

Perform the following exercises twice per day to improve strength of individual core muscles.

Posterior Pelvic Tilt

Lie on your back with your knees bent. Tighten and suck in your stomach and press your low back into the floor. Think about drawing your belly button inward toward your spine. Hold for a count of three, then relax for a second; repeat twenty times.

Bridge

Lie on your back with your knees bent. Tighten your buttock muscles and raise your hips off the floor, then lower your hips back down; repeat twenty times using a slow, controlled motion.

Crunch

Lie on your back with your knees bent. Support your neck with a towel. Contract your stomach muscles to lift your shoulders off the floor a few inches, then lower. Repeat this twenty times using a slow, controlled motion.

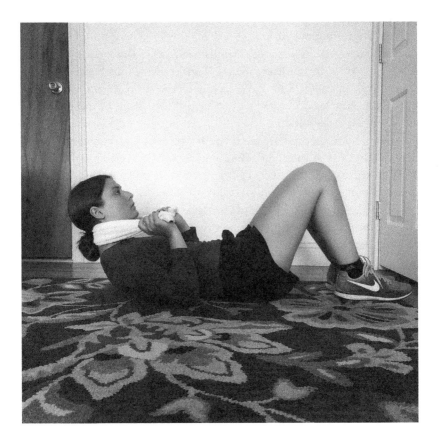

Clamshell

Lie on your side with your knees bent. Keep your feet together and raise your top knee (like a clamshell opening), then lower the knee; repeat twenty times using a slow, controlled motion. Do not roll your hips back. Repeat on your other side.

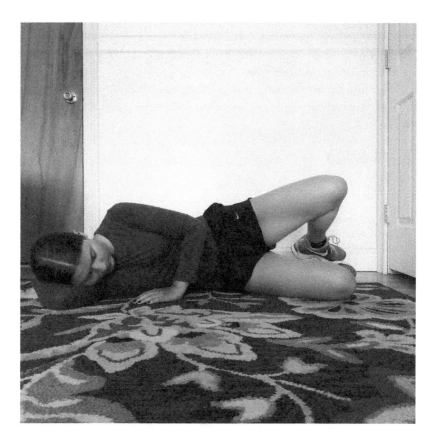

RESTORE NORMAL MOVEMENT PATTERNS

The following exercises improve core strength as well, but they also force your muscles to work together in a coordinated fashion, or synergy. Improved synergy carries over to everyday activities and helps normalize movement patterns.

Do not try these exercises before you are ready. The exercises should challenge you, but you should not have to struggle to keep your balance. Adequate flexibility and strength of isolated movements are necessary to progress to this stage. Your therapist can help you determine the appropriate time to progress.

Because there are many muscles that control both your low back and hips, you will recognize many of the following exercises from chapter 17.

Perform the following exercises twice per day to improve movement patterns.

Quadruped Opposite Arm/Leg Lift

On all fours, simultaneously lift your right arm and left leg up to a horizontal position. Lower and repeat with your left arm and right leg.

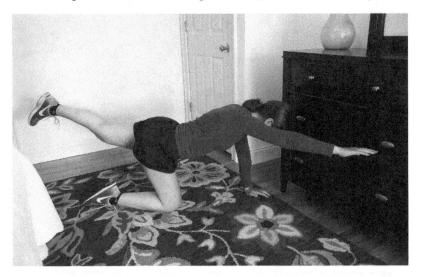

Repeat this twenty times using a slow, controlled motion. Try to keep your low back as still as possible. Imagine a hot cup of coffee sitting on your low back; you don't want it to spill!

Standing Hip Abduction

Stand and rest your hands on a table or countertop for balance. Raise one leg to the side, then let it back down; repeat twenty times using a slow, controlled motion. Repeat with your other leg. Keep your foot pointing straight ahead and don't raise your leg too high. When this becomes easy, tie a stretch band around your ankles to provide resistance.

Standing Hip Extension

Stand and rest your hands on a table or countertop for balance. Raise one leg back with your knee straight, then let it back down; repeat twenty times using a slow, controlled motion. Repeat with your other leg. When this becomes easy, tie a stretch band around your ankles to provide resistance.

Side Step

Stand with your knees slightly bent and sidestep across the room for twenty steps, then back the other way for twenty steps. Keep your feet pointing straight ahead. When this becomes easy, tie a stretch band around your ankles to provide resistance.

Mini-Squat

Stand with your feet shoulder width apart. Rest your hands on a table or countertop for balance. Keep your back straight, squat down part way, then return to standing; repeat twenty times using a slow, controlled motion.

Short Lunge

Stand with your feet shoulder width apart. Keep your back straight and step forward with one leg to the position shown. Push back to the starting position and repeat with your other leg. Continue to alternate legs and complete ten on each leg using a slow, controlled motion.

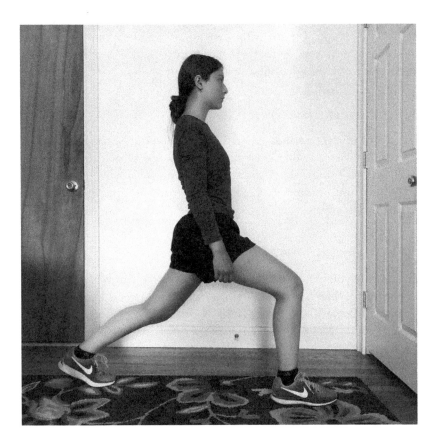

Single-Leg Balance

Balance on one leg and count to ten, then rest for a few seconds; repeat ten times. Repeat with the other leg. Touch a table or wall lightly if needed to keep from falling.

Single-Leg Balance with Leg Swings

Balance on one leg and swing your other leg forward and back twenty times, then swing it side to side across the front of your body twenty times. Repeat on the other leg. Touch a table or wall lightly if needed to keep from falling.

19

NECK INJURIES

A treatment method called blood flow restriction training, or BFR, is gaining popularity in gyms and physical therapy clinics. This technique employs a tourniquet that restricts blood flow to muscles during exercise. This stresses the muscles, which respond by getting stronger. Research shows that this technique increases production of many cellular components of muscle growth, which can result in more rapid strength gains than traditional strength training produces. BFR is particularly beneficial after surgery, when traditional strengthening can be slow and difficult.[1]

I would like to take this opportunity to mention how proud I am to be a member of a profession that is filled with people who wake up in the morning with ideas like, "I think I'll see what happens if I put a tourniquet around my leg while I exercise today."

I would also like to point out a safety precaution that I haven't run across in the literature on blood flow restriction training. If you remember my rant in the last chapter over the danger of hanging upside down for too long, you may see where this is going, so I'll just make it short and simple: Don't use blood flow restriction training on your neck. This could lead to death. (I also don't recommend it for treating erectile dysfunction.)

A much safer way to treat neck injuries involves the same four objectives described earlier—decrease the body's response, restore normal range of motion, restore normal strength, and restore normal movement patterns—while following restrictions your physician imposes. The structure of your neck is basically the same as your low back, with smaller parts, so everything I said in the last chapter regarding MRI images and radicular symptoms applies to your neck as well. The only

165

important difference is that radicular symptoms from your neck occur in your shoulders, arms, and hands instead of your hips, legs, and feet.

DECREASE THE BODY'S RESPONSE

Neck muscles are postural muscles, so they are prone to fierce spasm that can worsen if you try to force motion. So if you move the wrong way and strain your neck, follow the same procedure I described for your low back. Don't move. Relax. Breathe. Find a comfortable position, stay there for a few minutes, then move out of it slowly. Don't run around bending and twisting and pulling on your neck. Use ice or heat or both. Wait a day before starting exercises.

RESTORE NORMAL FLEXIBILITY

Even though your neck is similar to your low back, rehabilitation is very different. As I described in chapter 18, the best way to use your low back is to hold your back relatively still and perform most of the motions with your legs. So low back rehabilitation involves more leg stretching and less back stretching. This does not apply to your neck, because most normal activities require good neck flexibility. Try driving to work without turning your head and you'll see what I mean.

Your neck, or cervical spine, moves in four directions: flexion (forward bend), extension (backward bend), lateral flexion (side bend), and rotation (twist).

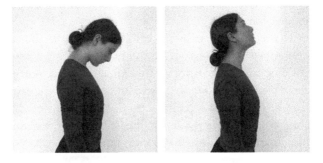

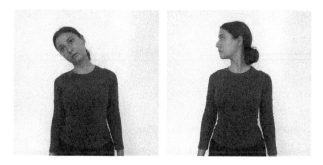

You have several layers of neck muscles: large outer muscles cover progressively smaller, deeper muscles. Many of these muscles travel up your neck and attach to the base of your skull, so spasm or tightness often causes headaches. Spasm can also be very tender to touch, and many patients say, "It feels like there's a rock in there." Gentle stretching can relieve this spasm and restore normal motion.

Perform the following exercises twice per day to improve neck flexibility.

Side Bending Stretch

To stretch your right side, sit on a chair and hold the chair with your right hand. (This keeps your right shoulder from lifting up.) With your left hand, pull your head to the left. Hold the stretch and count to ten, then return to the start position for a second; repeat this ten times. You should feel a stretch on the right side of your head, neck, or shoulder. Stop if you feel pain on the left side of your head, neck, or shoulder. Stop if you feel increased radicular symptoms down either side. Repeat on the other side.

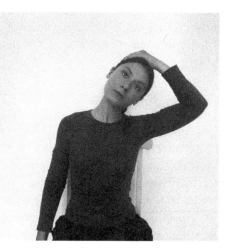

Forward Side Bending Stretch

To stretch your right side, sit on a chair and hold the chair with your right hand. (This keeps your right shoulder from lifting up.) With your left hand, pull your head to the left and to the front (about halfway between left and front). Hold the stretch and count to ten, then return to the start position for a second; repeat this ten times. You should feel a stretch on the right side of your head, neck, or shoulder, but a little 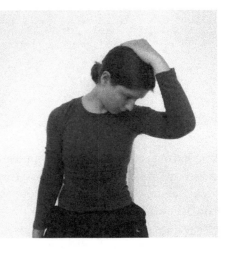 more in toward your spine. Stop if you feel pain on the left side of your head, neck, or shoulder. Stop if you feel increased radicular symptoms down either side. Repeat on the other side.

Cervical Rotation Stretch

Sit or stand straight with good posture. Keep your shoulders still and rotate your head to the right. Hold the stretch and count to ten, then rotate your head to the left and hold the stretch for a count of ten. Repeat this ten times. Stop if you feel increased radicular symptoms down either side.

Corner Stretch

Muscle spasm from a neck injury can pull your shoulders forward and create poor posture, also known as forward-head, rounded-shoulders posture. This posture can cause the muscles in the front of your shoulders and chest to become tight. Perform the following exercise twice per day to improve flexibility of these muscles.

Stand facing a corner with both arms up on the walls, your elbows the same height as your shoulders, and your elbows bent to 90 degrees.

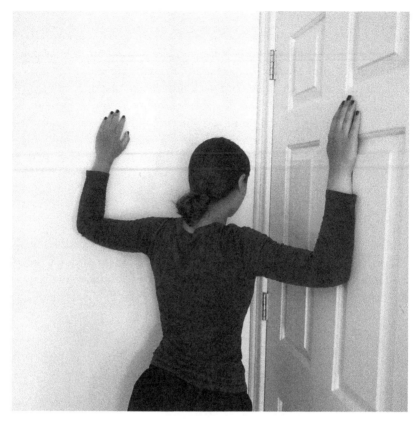

Lean your body into the corner, hold for a count of ten, then relax for a second; repeat ten times. You should feel a stretch in the front of your shoulders or chest. Stop if you feel increased radicular symptoms.

RESTORE NORMAL STRENGTH

It is important to strengthen your neck muscles, but it is even more important to improve your posture. Poor posture puts the structures in your neck into prolonged unnatural positions, which creates wear and tear and chronic pain. Pull one of your fingers back the wrong direction and hold it there for a few minutes. Hurts, right? This is what poor posture does to your neck.

Poor posture can result from a neck injury or it can cause a neck injury. Either way, you must achieve two main objectives to correct your posture: strengthen the postural muscles and retrain the subconscious part of your brain to break the poor posture habit.

Postural muscles include your neck muscles and the muscles in your upper back between your shoulder blades, or interscapular muscles. If you are in a poor postural position while strengthening these muscles, the exercises will only reinforce your poor posture, so you must maintain correct posture during exercises. The best way to do this is with a movement called the chin tuck.

Chin Tuck

In a sitting or standing position, tuck your chin in toward your neck by gliding your head straight back. Do not tilt your head up or down; keep it straight. When you put your head in the correct position, the rest of the cervical spine falls into the correct position as well.

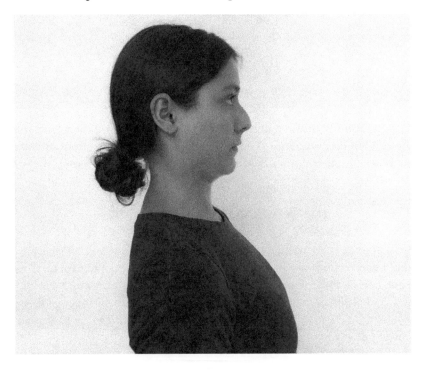

To use this movement as an exercise, hold the position for a count of ten, relax, and repeat ten times. This exercise can be done anywhere: sitting at your desk, standing in line, stopped at a red light. Perform this exercise several times throughout the day.

To use this movement to maintain correct posture during exercise, simply perform the chin tuck and hold it for the duration of the exercise.

You must be careful when you strengthen your neck muscles. Many people injure their necks performing exercises that involve pushing heavy weights through excessive ranges of motion. The safest way to strengthen your neck is to perform isometric exercises, which involve no motion and are done with your neck held in a neutral position.

Perform the following isometric exercises twice per day to improve strength of your neck muscles.

Isometric Cervical Flexion

Assume the chin tuck position and place the fingers of both hands on your forehead. Without moving, push your head into your fingers. Do not push as hard as you can. Instead push with about 50 percent of your maximal effort and hold for a count of ten, then relax for a second; repeat ten times. Stop if you feel a sharp pain or radicular symptoms.

Isometric Cervical Extension

Assume the chin tuck position and place the fingers of both hands on the back of your head. Without moving, push your head into your fingers. Do not push as hard as you can. Rather, push with about 50 percent of your maximal effort and hold for a count of ten, then relax for a second; repeat ten times. Stop if you feel a sharp pain or radicular symptoms.

Isometric Cervical Side Bending

Assume the chin tuck position and place the fingers of one hand on the side of your head. Without moving, push your head into your fingers. Do not push as hard as you can. Instead, push with about 50 percent of your maximal effort and hold for a count of ten, then relax for a second;

repeat ten times. Stop if you feel a sharp pain or radicular symptoms. Repeat on the other side.

Although isometric exercises are effective for interscapular strengthening, isotonic exercises, or exercises involving movements, are also safe because they involve movements of your shoulders, not your neck. Perform the following exercises twice per day to improve strength of your interscapular muscles.

Scapular Retraction

Assume the chin tuck position. Squeeze your shoulder blades together, hold for a count of ten, then relax for a second; repeat ten times.

Prone Shoulder Abduction

Lie on your stomach, lift your head, and assume the chin tuck position. With your arms straight out, palms down, lift and lower your arms using a slow, controlled motion; repeat twenty times.

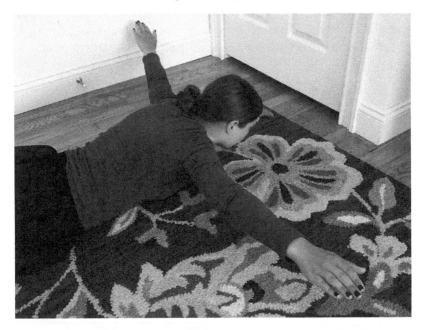

Prone Shoulder Extension

Lie on your stomach, lift your head, and assume the chin tuck position. With the arms at your side, palms up, lift and lower your arms using a slow, controlled motion; repeat twenty times.

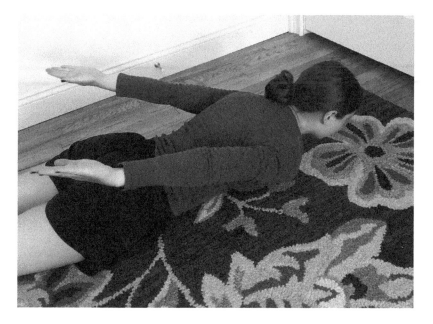

RESTORE NORMAL MOVEMENT PATTERNS

Maintaining good posture during all activities is the most important aspect of proper movement of the cervical spine. Strength is not nearly as important as habit. You could have the strongest postural muscles in the world and still fall back into poor posture when you stop thinking about it. One way to change this habit is to incorporate the chin tuck into every exercise in your program. Even your leg exercises. Whatever exercise routine you follow, assume the chin tuck position to begin each exercise. Repetition is the only way to change a habit.

You can also incorporate this repetition into your daily life by setting your alarm to vibrate every hour. This will remind you to assume the chin tuck position and hold it for as long as you remember to hold it. This is not physically demanding. When your head is back, it is more balanced over your spine. When your head is forward, more neck muscle contraction is needed to keep your head from falling forward.

You may have heard that the best way to correct your posture is to pull your shoulders back. This will correct your posture, but it takes more muscular effort and you will fatigue. In the chin tuck position, your shoulders come back automatically.

20

SHOULDER INJURIES

The shoulder is the most complex joint in the body. The term "shoulder joint" is actually incorrect. A more accurate term is "shoulder joint complex," because the shoulder is made up of four joints: the glenohumeral joint (between the arm and the shoulder blade), the scapulothoracic joint (between the shoulder blade and the rib cage), the acromioclavicular joint (between the shoulder blade and the collarbone), and the sternoclavicular joint (between the collarbone and the breastbone). All of these joints move, and the combination of all of these motions gives the shoulder more range of motion in more directions than any other joint.

To allow for these motions, shoulder ligaments are very loose—too loose, in fact, to hold the joint together, so the shoulder is held together by four muscles that are collectively called the rotator cuff. As I mentioned briefly in chapter 9, the rotator cuff is made up of four deep muscles that run along the shoulder blade and attach to the top of the arm bone. If the rotator cuff muscles become paralyzed by a stroke, the shoulder will fall out of joint and dislocate. This will not happen to any other joint in the body.

Another unique feature of the rotator cuff is that it is the most mispronounced term in the history of human anatomy. It is pronounced incorrectly even more often than terms like "osteochondritis of the tibial tubercle." Patients frequently tell me that they tore their rotary cup. So I want to clear something up right now. There is no such thing as a rotary cup. There is also no such thing as a rotor cusp, rotation crust, or radial crup. It's *ro-ta-tor-cuff*. If you get this right, you're halfway to recovery, and your therapist will love you forever.

Shoulders are notorious for becoming painful or tight, or both, with no traumatic injury, and this often becomes worse if not treated.

So if your shoulder starts to bother you for no apparent reason, do not hope that it gets better. Get it checked. As with all other body parts, you must follow your doctor's restrictions while you work on the four objectives—decrease the body's response, restore normal range of motion, restore normal strength, and restore normal movement patterns.

DECREASE THE BODY'S RESPONSE

Shoulders are particularly susceptible to inflammation that spirals out of control and causes extreme tightness and pain. This condition is called adhesive capsulitis, or frozen shoulder. Adhesive capsulitis can occur after surgery, after an injury, or out of the blue with no traumatic event. Most people instinctively protect and stop using their shoulders at the first sign of pain or tightness. This is exactly the wrong thing to do, because the more a frozen shoulder is *not* moved, the tighter it will get. The best way to decrease inflammation is with gentle early motion. So once every hour, perform the following three exercises.

Forward Pendulum Swing

Lean forward with your good arm resting on a table or countertop. Swing your painful arm gently to the front, just to the point where you feel a light stretch, then let it swing back down; repeat twenty times using a slow, controlled motion.

Side Pendulum Swing

Lean forward with your good arm resting on a table or countertop. Swing your painful arm gently to the side, just to the point where you feel a light stretch, then let it swing back down; repeat twenty times using a slow, controlled motion.

Elbow Flare

Hold your hands behind your head and gently bring your elbows in and out twenty times using a slow controlled motion. If this exercise causes sharp, severe pain, perform the forearm flare instead.

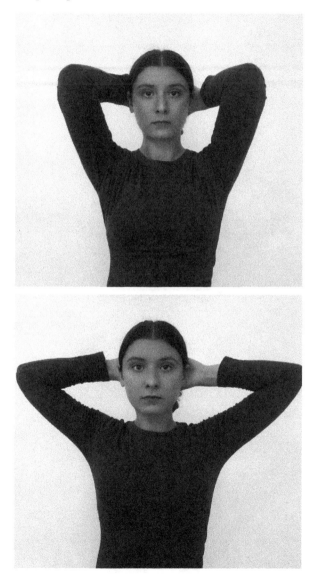

Forearm Flare

With your arms at your sides and your elbows bent to ninety degrees, keep your elbows at your sides and rotate your arms out and back twenty times using a slow controlled motion.

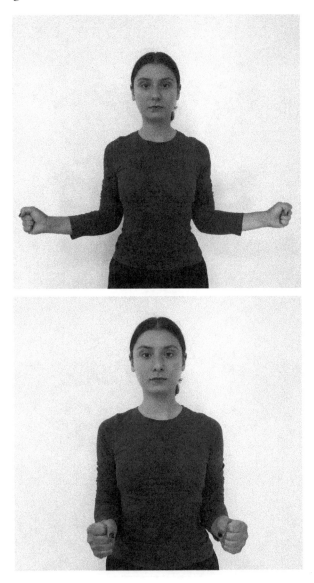

In addition to performing these exercises once every hour, apply ice for ten minutes, two or three times per day, and that is the treatment for inflammation.

RESTORE NORMAL FLEXIBILITY

Do not wait until inflammation subsides before you work on flexibility. Start right away. The most common complication after a shoulder injury or surgery is tightness, and the earlier you work on flexibility, the better. Old medical literature purported that frozen shoulders "thawed out" if rested for several months or even years. If you read or hear this, I want you to remember one thing: It is hogwash. I have never seen, and I have never spoken to a doctor who has ever seen, a shoulder that miraculously recovered normal motion after resting for months or years, and current research shows that frozen shoulders do not recover if they are ignored.[1]

The most important part of shoulder stretching is the location of where you feel the stretch. If you feel pain in the wrong place, you will irritate the inflamed tissue, and this will not improve motion. So when you perform the following exercises, pay close attention to the descriptions of where you should feel the stretch, and where you should not feel pain.

The four motions of your shoulder are flexion, abduction, external rotation, and internal rotation.

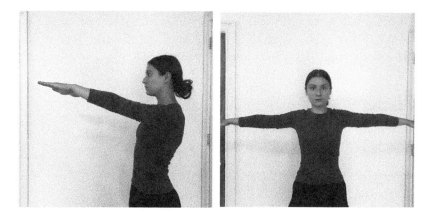

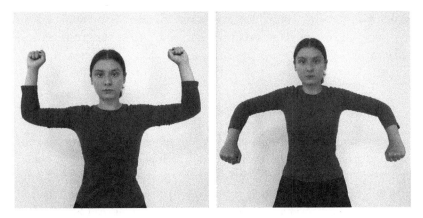

If you have a hard time reaching the back of your head to wash or brush your hair, you have limited external rotation. If you have a hard time reaching behind you to pull up your pants or reach your back pocket, you have limited internal rotation.

Perform the following exercises twice per day to improve shoulder flexion.

Flexion Table Slide

Sit in front of a table a foot or two away from the table. Place your hand on the table directly in front of you with your elbow straight. Lean forward and slide your hand forward on the table. You may want to place your hand on a small towel to help it slide easier. Hold for a count of ten, then slide your hand back toward you; repeat this ten times. You should feel a stretch in your armpit or back of your shoulder. Stop if you feel a sharp pain in the front or top of your shoulder.

Sink Flexion Stretch

Holding the edge of a sink or something sturdy, bend forward and step back to stretch your arm over your head. Hold for a count of ten, then relax for a second; repeat ten times. You should feel a stretch in your armpit or back of your shoulder. Stop if you feel a sharp pain in the front or top of your shoulder.

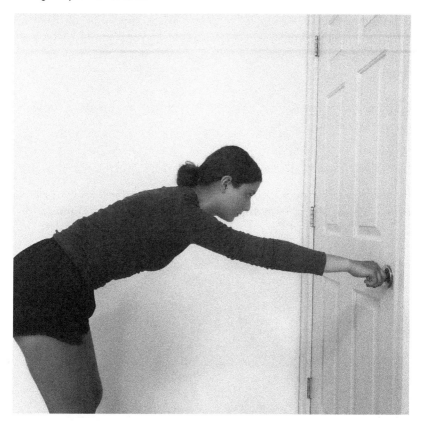

Flexion Hang

Grab the top of a door jamb or the top of a refrigerator with both hands shoulder width apart. Keep your shoulders relaxed and bend your knees to lower your body. Hold for a count of ten, then relax for a second; repeat ten times. You should feel a stretch in your armpit or back of your shoulder. Stop if you feel a sharp pain in the front or top of your shoulder.

Supine Cane Flexion

Lie on your back and hold something like a cane or yardstick with your hands shoulder width apart. Keep your elbows straight and lift your arms overhead. Hold for a count of ten, then lower your arms all the way; repeat ten times. You should feel a stretch in your armpit or back of your shoulder. Stop if you feel a sharp pain in the front or top of your shoulder.

Perform the following exercises twice per day to improve shoulder external rotation.

Table External Rotation Stretch

Sit next to a table and rest your painful arm on the table with your elbow bent at a right ankle. Lean your body forward, hold for a count of ten,

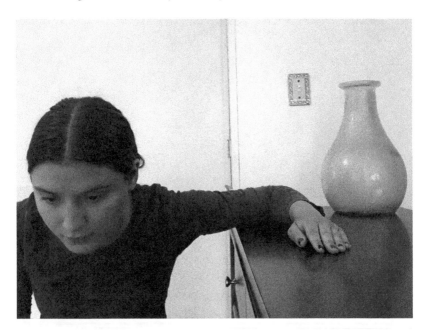

then rest for a second; repeat ten times. You should feel a stretch in the front of your shoulder or chest. Stop if you feel a sharp pain in the back of your shoulder.

Supine Cane External Rotation

Lie on your back and hold something like a cane or yardstick with your elbows bent at right angles. Rotate the cane over your head, hold for a count of ten, then return to the starting position; repeat ten times. You should feel a stretch in the front of your shoulder or chest. Stop if you feel a sharp pain in the back of your shoulder.

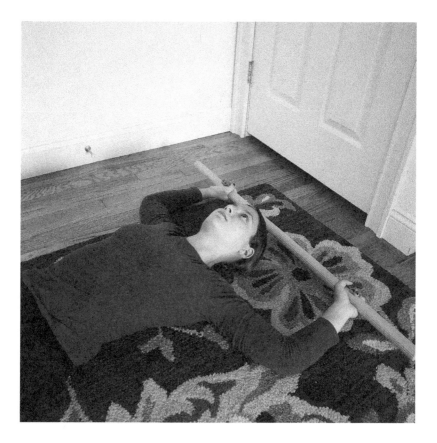

Corner Stretch

Stand facing a corner with both arms up on the walls, your elbows the same height as your shoulders, and your elbows bent to 90 degrees. Lean your body into the corner, hold for a count of ten, then relax for a second; repeat ten times. You should feel a stretch in the front of your shoulder or chest. Stop if you feel a sharp pain in the back of your shoulder.

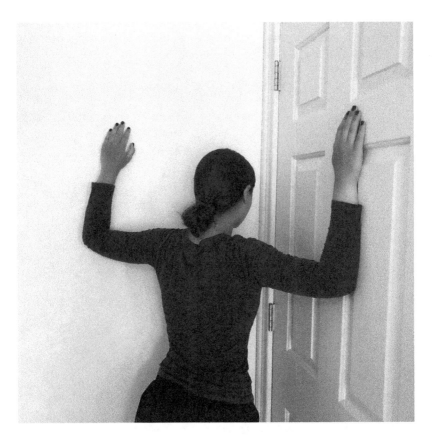

Perform the following exercises twice per day to improve shoulder internal rotation.

Side-Lying Internal Rotation Stretch

Lie on your painful shoulder with your arm to the front and your elbow bent to 90 degrees. Use your other hand to push your forearm toward the floor, hold for a count of ten, then return to the starting position; repeat ten times. Your body weight should keep your shoulder from rolling up. If you push your arm all the way to the floor, you are probably rolling your shoulder up, so try to center your bodyweight directly over your shoulder. You should feel a stretch in the back or top of your shoulder or upper arm. Stop if you feel a sharp pain in the front of your shoulder.

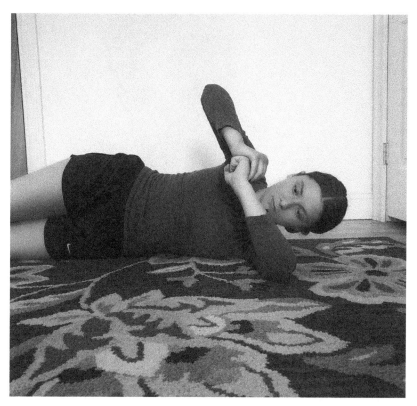

Behind-the-Back Towel Stretch

Place your painful arm behind your back at waist level. Place your other hand behind your head. Hold the ends of a towel in each hand. Keep your painful arm relaxed and use your other arm to pull your painful arm up the middle of your back. Hold for a count of ten, return to the starting position, and repeat ten times. Keep your shoulders back—do not roll them forward. You should feel a stretch in the back or top of your shoulder or upper arm. Stop if you feel a sharp pain in the front of your shoulder.

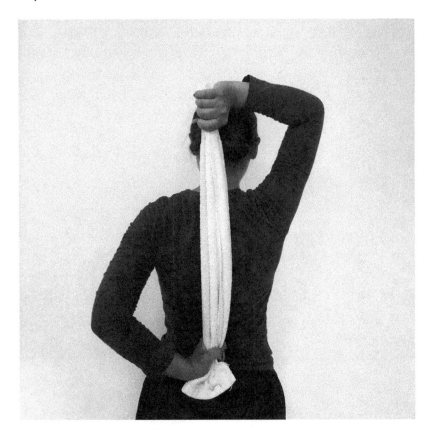

RESTORE NORMAL STRENGTH

If your shoulder is tight, don't start strengthening until you have performed a week or two of stretching. I am not aware of any research that supports or refutes this advice. I base it on my own experience treating thousands of people with shoulder injuries and my observation that if they attempted strengthening before restoring some flexibility, most of them experienced flare-ups of inflammation. Tight shoulders do not move properly, and strengthening exercises can actually reinforce improper movements and create more wear and tear.

Shoulder muscles can be described as belonging to either of two main groups: large outer muscles and small deep muscles. The large outer muscles move the arm. The small deep muscles hold the joint together and keep the joint congruent during these motions. As I described at the beginning of this chapter, the small deep muscles are collectively called the rotator cuff. When the large outer muscles lift the arm, the rotator cuff actually pulls *down* on the head of the humerus (top of the arm bone). If it weren't for this downward pull, the shoulder would hike up during elevation. People with large rotator cuff tears exhibit this motion.

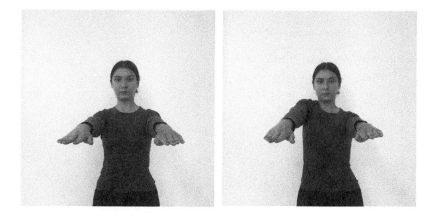

If the small deep muscles of the rotator cuff are weak, your shoulder will not move properly, so it is important to strengthen these muscles first. Perform the following exercises twice per day to improve strength of your rotator cuff.

Stretch Band External Rotation

Bend your elbow to 90 degrees, hold your elbow at your side, use a stretch band to provide resistance, and rotate your arm outward. Return to the start position and repeat twenty times using a slow, controlled motion. Do not straighten your elbow or move your elbow away from your body—these are the two most common mistakes.

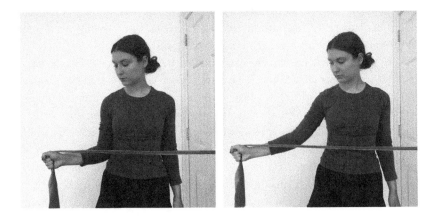

Stretch Band Internal Rotation

Bend your elbow to 90 degrees, hold your elbow at your side, use a stretch band to provide resistance, and rotate your arm inward. Return to the start position and repeat twenty times using a slow, controlled motion.

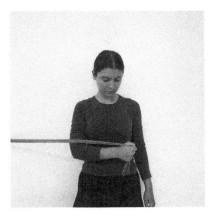

Side-Lying External Rotation

Lie on your side with your injured shoulder up. Bend your elbow to 90 degrees, hold your elbow at your side, and rotate your arm outward. Return to the start position and repeat twenty times using a slow, controlled motion. Use a light weight or soup can to provide resistance. Do not straighten your elbow or move your elbow away from your body.

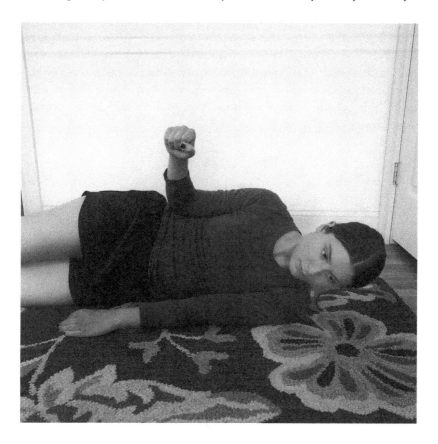

Once your rotator cuff has gained some strength, you can start to strengthen your large outer muscles. Perform the following exercises twice per day to improve strength of these muscles.

Standing Shoulder Flexion

Stand in front of a full-length mirror. With your palms down, lift your arms in front of you to shoulder level and no higher. Watch your shoulders in the mirror and make sure you do not hike your injured shoulder. If you cannot keep your shoulder from hiking, lift your arms only to the height that you can perform without hiking. Return to the start position and repeat twenty times using a slow, controlled motion. When this becomes easy, hold soup cans or light weights to provide minor resistance.

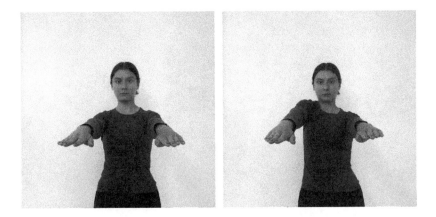

Standing Shoulder Abduction

Stand in front of a full-length mirror. With your thumbs up, lift your arms to the side to shoulder level and no higher. Watch your shoulders in the mirror and make sure you do not hike your injured shoulder. If you cannot keep your shoulder from hiking, lift your arms only to the height that you can perform without hiking. Return to the start position and repeat twenty times using a slow, controlled motion. When

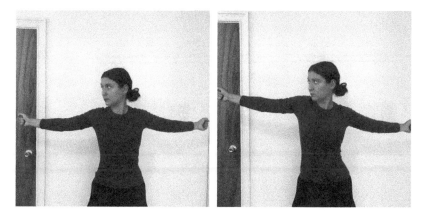

this becomes easy, hold soup cans or light weights to provide gentle resistance.

RESTORE NORMAL MOVEMENT PATTERNS

If your shoulder is tight or weak, your body will alter the way it moves in order to get the job done. You will unconsciously hike your shoulder or roll it forward or backward in order to reach what you need to reach. These abnormal movements can turn into habits and persist even after you have restored adequate strength and range of motion. To correct abnormal movements, you need to first see them. Stand in front of a mirror and watch yourself raise both arms straight up over your head, then up to the side, then behind your head, then down behind your low back. You can try other motions as well. Use your imagination. Look for any motion of your injured side that looks different from the same motion of your uninjured side and practice those motions in front of the mirror. Try to make the motions of your injured side match the motions of your uninjured side. Pay attention to how you move throughout the day and apply what you learn from this exercise. Repetition of proper movements is the only way to break bad habits.

21

ELBOW INJURIES

Elbow injuries tend to have creative nicknames like tennis elbow, golfer's elbow, and nursemaid's elbow. But I have noticed something odd over the years. Of all the patients I have treated for tennis elbow, almost none of them played tennis. Same goes for golfer's elbow. I don't think I've ever met an actual nursemaid, so I'm not sure about that one, but the point is, I'm beginning to think that whoever came up with these names was probably the same comedian who picked the term "reducing" to mean popping a joint back into place.

In my experience, people who develop elbow pain are typically mechanics, carpenters, plumbers, electricians, and others who do a lot of heavy or repetitive twisting motions with their hands and forearms. Those who do a lot of vacuuming, knitting or needlepoint, typing, or computer work are also prone to elbow pain. So rest assured that if you are not in these groups, you can play all the golf and tennis you want and go hog wild with nursemaiding activities, and you still have a relatively low chance of developing elbow pain.

Most of the forearm muscles attach to the inside or outside of the elbow and travel down to control motions of the wrist and hand. The muscles that attach to the inside of the elbow (medial epicondyle) act to flex the wrist, bend the fingers, and rotate the forearm to a palm-down position. The muscles that attach to the outside of the elbow (lateral epicondyle) act to extend the wrist, straighten the fingers, and rotate the forearm to a palm-up position.

The above-mentioned conditions are defined as follows: Golfer's elbow is an inflammation of the tendons that attach to the medial epicondyle, tennis elbow is an inflammation of the tendons that attach to the lateral epicondyle, and nursemaid's elbow is a partial dislocation caused by a sudden pull that often happens to young children when their parents (or nursemaids) yank their arms to get them out of traffic. (For once I am not joking. That is really how nursemaid's elbow got its name.)

Whether you sustain an elbow injury or have pain that came on with no traumatic event, follow your doctor's restrictions as you work on the four objectives that should be burned into your memory by now: decrease the body's response, restore normal range of motion, restore normal strength, and restore normal movement patterns.

DECREASE THE BODY'S RESPONSE

The tendons that attach to the elbow are vulnerable to inflammation because many people perform repetitive motions over and over without adequate recovery time. If inflammation is not dealt with, it can travel down to the forearm muscles, which can become tight, swollen, tender, and very painful. Don't ignore this pain and push through it. If left untreated, inflammation can become chronic, and tissue layers that normally glide on each other can adhere into a solid mass. Inflamed tissues that have reached this point will likely not respond to physical therapy, ice, medications, or even injections, and surgery may be needed to cut the adhesions and separate the tissue layers.

As with all body parts, early gentle motion is the best treatment for inflammation. Perform the following two exercises once every hour.

Wrist Flexion/Extension

With your elbow bent to 90 degrees and your thumb up, make a loose fist and bend your wrist in and out twenty times using a slow, controlled motion.

Forearm Pronation/Supination

With your elbow bent to 90 degrees and your hand flat, turn your palm up, then down; repeat twenty times using a slow, controlled motion.

Elbow pain usually occurs in a small area, so the best way to ice is to hold an ice cube in your other hand (with a towel, so you don't freeze your fingers) and rub the ice right on the painful spot. Keep the ice moving in circles—if you hold it still you can freeze your skin—and do this for five minutes, two or three times per day.

RESTORE NORMAL FLEXIBILITY

The most important structures to stretch are the forearm muscles, more specifically, the wrist flexors and extensors. Perform the following exercise twice per day to stretch the wrist flexors.

Wrist Flexor Stretch

Hold your painful arm straight out with your palm up. Use your other hand to stretch your wrist downward. Hold the stretch for a count of

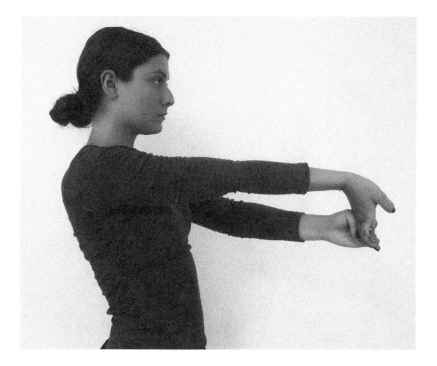

ten, then relax for a second; repeat ten times. You should feel a stretch in the palm side of your forearm or the inside of your elbow. You may feel some pain on the outside of your elbow; this is okay, but stop or pull more gently if this pain is severe. Stop or bend your elbow slightly if you feel pain in the back of your elbow.

Wrist Extensor Stretch

Perform the following exercise twice per day to stretch the wrist extensors.

Hold your painful arm straight out with your palm down. Use your other hand to pull your wrist down. Hold the stretch for a count of ten, then relax for a second; repeat ten times. You should feel a stretch in

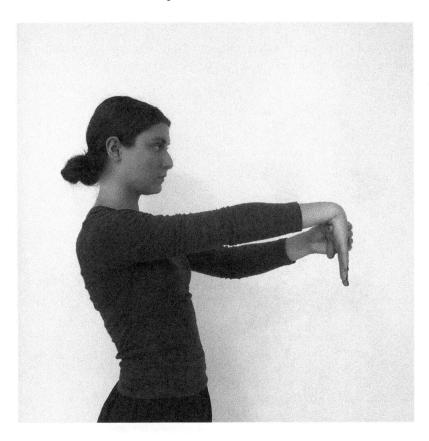

the outside of your forearm or elbow. You may feel some pain on the inside of your elbow; this is okay, but stop or pull more gently if this pain is severe.

RESTORE NORMAL STRENGTH

To avoid flaring up inflammation, don't start strengthening until you have performed two or three days of stretching. Moderate pain is okay during strengthening, but stop or lighten the weight if you experience sharp or severe pain.

Perform the following exercises twice per day to strengthen the wrist and forearm.

Wrist Curl

Rest your forearm on your leg with your palm up. Hold a soup can or light weight and curl your wrist up, then down using a slow, controlled motion; repeat twenty times.

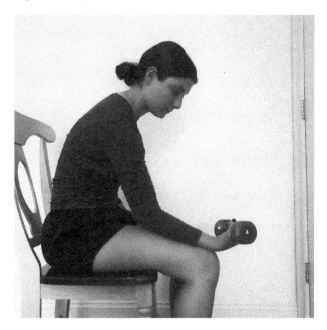

Reverse Wrist Curl

Rest your forearm on your leg with your palm down. Hold a soup can or light weight and curl your wrist up, then down using a slow, controlled motion; repeat twenty times.

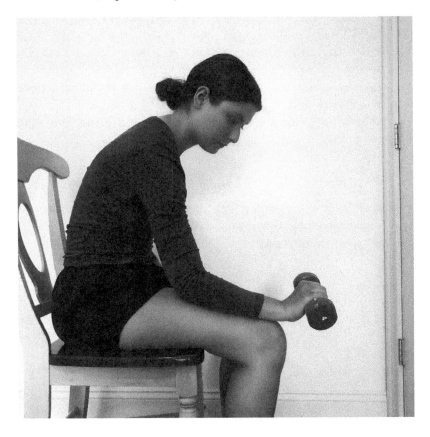

Hammer Pronation/Supination

Rest your forearm on your leg and hold the light end of a hammer with the heavy end pointing up. Turn your palm up to rotate the hammer until it is parallel with the floor, then turn your palm down to rotate the hammer until it is parallel with the floor. Repeat twenty times using a slow, controlled motion. If this is too difficult or causes severe pain, decrease the resistance by gripping the hammer closer to the heavy end.

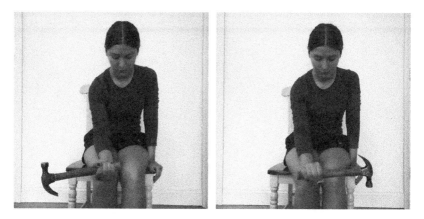

RESTORE NORMAL MOVEMENT PATTERNS

Elbow pain often leads to shoulder pain because of our old friend compensation. If your elbow is tight or weak, you may repetitively overwork or overstretch your shoulder to compensate for this. So use a mirror to follow the same procedure I described in chapter 20 to look for abnormal motions. Watch yourself raise both arms straight up over your head, then up to the side, then behind your head, then down behind your low back. Look for anything that is not symmetrical, and try to make the motions of your injured side match the motions of your uninjured side. Use repetition to create new habits.

22

WRIST AND HAND INJURIES

According to scientists, the structure of our hands is what separates us from other animals (besides hairpieces, coffee enemas, and mindfulness training), so hand injuries can be very complex. Physical and occupational therapists can take advanced training to become certified hand therapists, or CHTs. If you need hand therapy, do not go to a therapist who is not a CHT. Some hand injuries that seem relatively minor can lead to irreversible damage if not dealt with quickly and properly.

Since I am not a CHT, hand rehabilitation is outside my scope of practice, so I will not include a sample protocol. My apologies to those of you who suffered through this entire book hoping to learn how to rehabilitate your hands. The good news is that all of the principles I discussed for the rest of the body also apply to hands, so you can use your vast supply of newfound knowledge to impress your CHTs with the most intelligent and informed questions they have ever heard.

APPENDIX I

Strengthening for Those Who Hate Exercise

Since we have already established that you hate exercise, I'm going to assume that you don't have a universal exercise machine or a set of Olympic weights in your basement. That's fine. You do not need any of those things. There is one thing I will ask you to invest in: a gallon jug of water that you will use as a weight. As the weeks and months go by, strength training will cause an uncontrollable urge to check yourself out, so you may also want to invest in a full-length mirror.

This routine consists of three exercises that cover all of the major muscle groups. Perform the routine two times per week, never two days in a row.

BENT-OVER ROW

Assume the position shown at a sturdy coffee table or couch. Pull the gallon of water up to your waist using a slow, controlled rowing motion, then lower the same way. Do not swing the weight or twist your body. Perform as many as you can, rest for about fifteen seconds, and repeat on the other side. Repeat this cycle until you have performed four sets on each side.

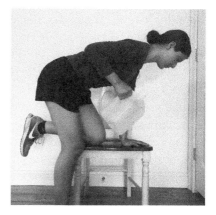

If you cannot perform at least ten on your first set, the weight is too heavy, so pour some of the water out. If you can perform fifty easily, look around for something heavier to use, or stop being so cheap and invest in some weights.

Rest for about one minute, then progress to the next exercise.

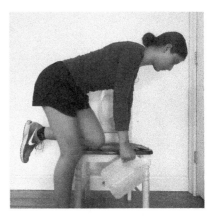

SQUAT

With your back straight, stomach tight, and feet shoulder width apart, squat down and then back up using a slow, controlled motion. Hold your arms straight out in front for balance. Do not bend your knees more than 90 degrees. Slowly do as many as you can using good form. Rest for about thirty seconds, then repeat. Do this until you have performed four sets.

It is okay for your heels to come up off the floor if this is more comfortable. It is also okay for your knees to come forward. You may hear some physical therapists warn that moving your knees forward will damage your knees. This is a myth that has not been supported by research.[1] Rest for about one minute, then progress to the next exercise.

PUSH-UP

Assume the push-up position with your hands a little wider than shoulder width apart. Perform a slow, controlled push-up, keeping your head up and lightly touching your chest to the floor. If you can't do ten, or even one, do them on your knees instead of your toes. Do as many as you can slowly with good form. Rest for about thirty seconds, then repeat. Do this until you have performed four sets.

WHAT TO EXPECT

You will probably be sore for the first few days. This is normal. If the soreness is severe, wait until it subsides before working out again. As always, stop if you feel sharp or severe pain. Proper diet and hydration are even more important during this stage than any other time.

Adjust this routine based on your fitness level. If four sets are too difficult, start with one or two sets. Increase the rest time between sets if necessary. Listen to your body.

When this routine becomes easy, you are ready to progress to the Jumbo Crossfit P90 XXX Suicide Bomber Edition workout.

APPENDIX II

Hormones

Hormone	Secreting Organ
adiponectin	adipose tissue
adrenocorticotropic hormone	anterior pituitary
aldosterone	adrenal cortex
amylin	pancreas
androstenedione	adrenal glands, gonads
angiotensin	liver
angiotensinogen	liver
antidiuretic hormone	posterior pituitary
anti–müllerian hormone	testes
atrial natriuretic peptide	heart
brain natriuretic peptide	heart
calcitonin	thyroid
cholecystokinin	duodenum
corticotropin–releasing hormone	hypothalamus
cortistatin	cerebral cortex
dehydroepiandrosterone	testes, ovary, kidney
dihydrotestosterone	multiple
endothelin	vascular endothelium
enkephalin	kidney
epinephrine	adrenal
erythropoietin	kidney
estrogen	ovary, testes

Hormone	Secreting Organ
follicle-stimulating hormone	anterior pituitary
galanin	CNS and GI tract
gastric inhibitory polypeptide	duodenum and jejunum
gastrin	stomach, duodenum
ghrelin	stomach
glucagon	pancreas
glucagon–like peptide–1	ilium
glucocorticoid	adrenal cortex
gonadotropin–releasing hormone	hypothalamus
growth hormone	anterior pituitary
growth hormone–releasing hormone	hypothalamus
guanylin	gut
hepcidin	liver
human chorionic gonadotropin	placenta
human placental lactogen	placenta
inhibin	testes, ovary, fetus
insulin	pancreas
insulin–like growth factor	liver
leptin	adipose tissue
leukotrienes	blood
lipotropin	anterior pituitary
luteinizing hormone	anterior pituitary
melanocyte-stimulating hormone	anterior pituitary / pars intermedia
melatonin	pineal
motilin	small intestine
norepinephrine	adrenal
orexin	hypothalamus
osteocalcin	skeleton
oxytocin	posterior pituitary

Hormone	Secreting Organ
pancreatic polypeptide	pancreas
parathyroid hormone	parathyroid gland
pituitary adenylate cyclase-activating peptide	multiple
progestogen	ovary, adrenal glands, placenta
prolactin	anterior pituitary, uterus
prolactin-releasing hormone	hypothalamus
prostacyclin	endothelium
prostaglandins	seminal vesicle
relaxin	ovary, uterus, placenta, mammary
renin	kidney
secosteroid	skin, kidneys
secretin	duodenum
somatostatin	hypothalamus, pancreas, GI tract
testosterone	testes, ovary
thrombopoietin	liver, kidney, striated muscle
thromboxane	blood
thyroid-stimulating hormone	anterior pituitary
thyrotropin-releasing hormone	hypothalamus
thyroxine	thyroid
triiodothyronine	thyroid
vasoactive intestinal peptide	pancreas, hypothalamus
uroguanylin	renal tissues

ACKNOWLEDGMENTS

I would like to sincerely thank all three readers who hung in there all the way to the end of this book. I apologize if you were looking for some basic first aid treatments for traumatic injuries involving broken bones. I would recommend going to the emergency room, but it's probably too late.

I would also like to apologize to all the physicians out there for making fun of your waiting room times. I assure you I was only kidding around. I did try to make up for this by recommending approximately four hundred times that people go to see their doctors. So, you're welcome.

Thank you to the thousands of patients who have shared their personal struggles and trusted me with their care. The opportunity to play a small part in so many lives has been a gift. Special thanks to Frank Ward for teaching me the meaning of determination and for letting me tell his story.

Thank you to all of the doctors, therapists, and other clinicians of many different disciplines who have worked with me over the years. I have learned more from you than from any book or journal.

Special thanks to my friends Matt Algeo, Bob Costello, and Susan Henderson, all accomplished authors who were more generous with their time and advice than I ever would have expected.

Huge thanks to my agent, Deborah Hofmann, for believing in this book and taking a chance on a first-time author. Her expertise, judgment, stamina, encouragement, sense of humor, and many, many hours of work helped me transform this book from an amateur first try into a literary masterpiece.

Thank you to my parents, Attila and Shirley Salamon, for having me, and for telling me how great this book was even after the first draft, which was pretty awful.

And above all, thanks to my wife, Melissa, and my daughters, Hannah, Katrina, and Kyra, for putting up with my constant dad jokes and for helping me bring this project to fruition.

I hope this book helped you understand the basics and improve your physical therapy experience. If you are interested in learning more details, keep an eye out for my future books. I will cover more specific injuries and techniques, including a new method for performing your own total knee replacement in the privacy of your own home using nothing but a set of Ginsu knives and a Dremel tool.

Until then, keep smiling.

NOTES

INTRODUCTION

1. Bradley Sawyer and Daniel McDermott, "How Does the Quality of the U.S. Healthcare System Compare to Other Countries?" *Peterson-KFF Health System Tracker*, March 28, 2019, https://www.healthsystemtracker.org/chart-collection/quality-u-s-healthcare-system-compare-countries/#item-start

2. Anthony Delitto et al., "Surgery versus Nonsurgical Treatment of Lumbar Spinal Stenosis: A Randomized Trial," *Annals of Internal Medicine* 162, no. 7 (April 7, 2015): 465–73, http://doi.org/10.7326/M14-1420.

3. Julie M. Fritz, Gerard P. Brennan, and Stephen J. Hunter, "Physical Therapy or Advanced Imaging as First Management Strategy Following a New Consultation for Low Back Pain in Primary Care: Associations with Future Health Care Utilization and Charges," *Health Services Research* 50, no. 6 (March 16, 2015): 1927–40, http://doi.org/10.1111/1475-6773.12301.

4. Bureau of Labor Statistics, "2016 Survey of Occupational Injuries and Illnesses Charts Package," November 9, 2017, https://www.bls.gov/iif/osch0060.pdf.

5. MedRisk 2018 Industry Trends Report, Physical Medicine and Workers' Comp, "Workers' Comp Costs: Why Physical Therapy Is Bigger Than You Think (Part 1 of 2)," https://www.medrisknet.com/workers-comp-costs-why-physical-therapy-is-bigger-than-you-think-part-1-of-2/.

6. Capstone Partners, Investment Banking Advisers, "Outpatient Physical Therapy, Q1 2017," https://capstoneheadwaters.com/sites/default/files/Capstone%20Outpatient%20Physical%20Therapy%20M&A%20Report_1Q%202017_0.pdf.

7. Munir J. Nasser, "How to Approach the Problem of Low Back Pain: An Overview," *Journal of Family and Community Medicine* 12, no. 1 (January–April 2005): 3–9, https://www.ncbi.nlm.nih.gov/pmc/articles/PMC3410134/?report=classic.

8. Lara Costa e Silva, Maria Isabel Fragoso, and Julia Teles, "Physical Activity-Related Injury Profile in Children and Adolescents according to Their Age, Maturation, and Level of Sports Participation," *Sports Health* 9, no. 2 (March–April 2017): 118–25, http://doi.org/10.1177/1941738116686964.

9. Yahtyng Sheu, Li-Hui Chen, and Holly Hedegaard, "Sports- and Recreation-Related Injury Episodes in the United States, 2011–2014," *National Health Statistics Reports* 99 (November 18, 2016): 1–12, https://pubmed.ncbi .nlm.nih.gov/27906643/.

10. Tareef Al-Aama, "Falls in the Elderly: Spectrum and Prevention," *Canadian Family Physician* 57, no. 7 (July 2011): 771–76, https://pubmed.ncbi.nlm .nih.gov/21753098/.

11. Mary Payne Bennett and Cecile Lengacher, "Humor and Laughter May Influence Health: III. Laughter and Health Outcomes," *Evidence-Based Complementary and Alternative Medicine* 5, no. 1 (March 2008): 37–40, https:// doi.org/10.1093/ecam/nem041.

CHAPTER 2

1. Arthur F. Kramer, Kirk I. Erickson, and Stanley J. Colcombe, "Exercise, Cognition, and the Aging Brain," *Journal of Applied Physiology* 101, no. 4 (October 2006): 1237–42, http://doi.org/10.1152/japplphysiol.00500.2006.

2. Kirk I. Erickson et al., "Exercise Training Increases Size of Hippocampus and Improves Memory," *Proceedings of the National Academy of Sciences of the United States of America* 108, no. 7 (February 15, 2011): 3017–22, http://doi .org/10.1073/pnas.1015950108.

3. Kirk I. Erickson, Regina L. Leckie, and Andrea M. Weinstein, "Physical Activity, Fitness, and Gray Matter Volume," *Neurobiology of Aging* 35, no. 2 (September 2014): S20–S28, http://doi.org/10.1016/j.neurobiolaging.2014.03.034.

CHAPTER 3

1. Aaron Stern, "Food Industry Influence on Dietary Advice in the United States," *Proceedings of the National Conference on Undergraduate Research*, April 7–9, 2016, University of North Carolina Asheville, https://www.coursehero.com/ file/44012761/1706-6525-1-PBpdf/.

2. Marion Nestle, "Food Lobbies, the Food Pyramid, and U.S. Nutrition Policy," *International Journal of Health Services* 23, no. 3 (July 1, 1993): 483–96, http://doi.org/10.2190/32F2-2PFB-MEG7-8HPU.

3. Michael Moss, *Salt, Sugar, Fat: How the Food Giants Hooked Us* (New York: Random House, 2013), xxv.

4. Nora D. Volkow et al., "Food and Drug Reward: Overlapping Circuits in Human Obesity and Addiction," *Current Topics in Behavioral Neurosciences* 11 (2012): 1–24, http://doi.org10.1007/7854_2011_169.

5. Shanna Swan et al., "Growth Hormones Fed to Beef Cattle Damage Human Health," *Organic Consumers Association*, May 1, 2007, https://www.organicconsumers.org/scientific/growth-hormones-fed-beef-cattle-damage-human-health.

6. Shanna Swan et al., "Semen Quality of Fertile US Males in Relation to Their Mother's Beef Consumption during Pregnancy," *Human Reproduction* 22, no. 6 (June 2007): 1497–502, http://doi.org/10.1093/humrep/dem068.

7. American Cancer Society, "Recombinant Bovine Growth Hormone," last modified September 10, 2014, https://www.cancer.org/cancer/cancer-causes/recombinant-bovine-growth-hormone.html.

8. Janice Tanne, "US Gets Mediocre Results Despite High Spending on Health Care," *British Medical Journal* 333, no. 7570 (September 30, 2006): 672, https://www.ncbi.nlm.nih.gov/pmc/articles/PMC1584360/.

9. Veronique Bouvard et al., "Carcinogenicity of Consumption of Red and Processed Meat," *Lancet Oncology* 16, no. 16 (December 2015): 1599–600, http://doi.org/10.1016/S1470-2045(15)00444-1.

10. Zeneng Wang et al., "Impact of Chronic Dietary Red Meat, White Meat, or Non-Meat Protein on Trimethylamine N-Oxide Metabolism and Renal Excretion in Healthy Men and Women," *European Heart Journal* 40, no. 7 (February 14, 2019): 583–94, http://doi.org/10.1093/eurheartj/ehy799.

11. David E. Andrich et al., "Relationship between Essential Amino Acids and Muscle Mass, Independent of Habitual Diets, in Pre- and Post-Menopausal US Women," *International Journal of Food Sciences and Nutrition* 62, no. 7 (November 2011): 719-24, http://doi.org/10.3109/09637486.2011.573772.

12. Ioannis Delimaris, "Adverse Effects Associated with Protein Intake above the Recommended Dietary Allowance for Adults," *ISRN Nutrition* (July 18, 2013): 126929, http://doi.org/10.5402/2013/126929.

13. Moamen Amin, Suganthiny Jeyaganth, and Armen Aprikian, "Dietary Habits and Prostate Cancer Detection: A Case-Control Study," *Canadian Urological Association Journal* 2, no. 5 (October 2008): 510–15, https://www.ncbi.nlm.nih.gov/pmc/articles/PMC2572247/#__ffn_sectitle.

14. Yan Song et al., "Whole Milk Intake Is Associated with Prostate Cancer–Specific Mortality among U.S. Male Physicians," *Journal of Nutrition* 143, no. 2 (February 2013): 189–96, http://doi.org/10.3945/jn.112.168484.

15. Xiang Gao, Michael P. LaValley, and Katherine L. Tucker, "Prospective Studies of Dairy Product and Calcium Intakes and Prostate Cancer Risk: A Meta-Analysis," *Journal of the National Cancer Institute* 97, no. 23 (December 7, 2005): 1768–77, http://doi.org/10.1093/jnci/dji402.

16. Susan E. McCann et al., "Usual Consumption of Specific Dairy Foods Is Associated with Breast Cancer in the Roswell Park Cancer Institute Databank and BioRepository," *Current Developments in Nutrition* 1, no. 3 (February 16, 2017): e000422, http://doi.org/10.3945/cdn.117.000422.

17. Susanna C. Larsson, Leif Bergkvist, and Alicja Wolk, "Milk and Lactose Intakes and Ovarian Cancer Risk in the Swedish Mammography Cohort," *American Journal of Clinical Nutrition* 80, no. 5 (November 2004): 1353–57, http://doi.org/10.1093/ajcn/80.5.1353.

18. Andreas Stang et al., "Adolescent Milk Fat and Galactose Consumption and Testicular Germ Cell Cancer," *Cancer Epidemiology, Biomarkers & Prevention* 15, no. 11 (November 2006): 2189–95, http://doi.org/10.1158/1055-9965.EPI-06-0372.

19. Mu Chen et al., "Dairy Fat and Risk of Cardiovascular Disease in 3 Cohorts of US Adults," *American Journal of Clinical Nutrition* 104, no. 5 (November 2016): 1209–17, http://doi.org/10.3945/ajcn.116.134460.

20. Frank B. Hu, "Plant-Based Foods and Prevention of Cardiovascular Disease: An Overview," *American Journal of Clinical Nutrition* 78, no. 3 (suppl) (September 2003): 544S–51S, http://doi.org/10.1093/ajcn/78.3.544S.

21. Diane Feskanich et al., "Milk, Dietary Calcium, and Bone Fractures in Women: A 12-Year Prospective Study," *American Journal of Public Health* 87, no. 6 (June 1997): 992–97, http://doi.org/10.2105/ajph.87.6.992.

22. Amy Joy Lanou, Susan E. Berkow, and Neal D. Barnard, "Calcium, Dairy Products, and Bone Health in Children and Young Adults: A Reevaluation of the Evidence," *Pediatrics* 115, no. 3 (March 2005): 736–43, http://doi.org/10.1542/peds.2004-0548.

23. Deborah E. Sellmeyer et al., "A High Ratio of Dietary Animal to Vegetable Protein Increases the Rate of Bone Loss and the Risk of Fracture in Postmenopausal Women," *American Journal of Clinical Nutrition* 73, no. 1 (January 2001): 118–22, http://doi.org/10.1093/ajcn/73.1.118.

24. Amy Joy Lanou, "Should Dairy be Recommended as Part of a Healthy Vegetarian Diet? Counterpoint," *American Journal of Clinical Nutrition* 89, no. 5 (May 2009): 1638S–42S, http://doi.org/10.3945/ajcn.2009.26736P.

25. Sanjay Basu et al., "The Relationship of Sugar to Population-Level Diabetes Prevalence: An Econometric Analysis of Repeated Cross-Sectional Data," *PLOS ONE* 8, no. 2 (February 27, 2013): e57873, http://doi.org/10.1371/journal.pone.0057873.

26. Robert H. Lustig, "Childhood Obesity: Behavioral Aberration or Biochemical Drive? Reinterpreting the First Law of Thermodynamics," *Nature Clinical Practice Endocrinology and Metabolism* 2, no. 8 (August 2006): 447–58, http://doi.org/10.1038/ncpendmet0220.

27. Yan Jiang et al., "A Sucrose-Enriched Diet Promotes Tumorigenesis in Mammary Gland in Part through the 12-Lipoxygenase Pathway," *Cancer Research* 76, no. 1 (January 1, 2016): 24–29, http://doi.org/10.1158/0008-5472.CAN-14-3432.

28. Quanhe Yang et al., "Added Sugar Intake and Cardiovascular Diseases Mortality among US Adults," *JAMA Internal Medicine* 174, no. 4 (April 2014): 516–24, http://doi.org/10.1001/jamainternmed.2013.13563.

29. David J. Jenkins et al., "Effect of a Very-High-Fiber Vegetable, Fruit, and Nut Diet on Serum Lipids and Colonic Function," *Metabolism* 50, no. 4 (April 2001): 494–503, http://doi.org/10.1053/meta.2001.21037.

30. Farin Kamangar and Ashkan Emadi, "Vitamin and Mineral Supplements: Do We Really Need Them?" *International Journal of Preventive Medicine* 3, no. 3 (March 2012): 221–26, https://pubmed.ncbi.nlm.nih.gov/22448315/.

31. Nisha Rao et al., "An Increase in Dietary Supplement Exposures Reported to US Poison Control Centers," *Journal of Medical Toxicology* 13, no. 3 (September 2017): 227–37, http://doi.org/10.1007/s13181-017-0623-7.

32. Theodore M. Brasky, Emily White, and Chi-Ling Chen, "Long-Term, Supplemental, One-Carbon Metabolism-Related Vitamin B Use in Relation to Lung Cancer Risk in the Vitamins and Lifestyle (VITAL) Cohort," *Journal of Clinical Oncology* 35, no. 30 (October 20, 2017): 3440–48, http://doi.org/10.1200/JCO.2017.72.7735.

33. Caldwell B. Esselstyn Jr. et al., "A Way to Reverse CAD?" *Journal of Family Practice* 63, no.7 (July 2014): 356–64b, https://pubmed.ncbi.nlm.nih.gov/25198208/.

CHAPTER 4

1. Goran Medic, Micheline Wille, and Michiel E. H. Hemels, "Short- and Long-Term Health Consequences of Sleep Disruption," *Nature and Science of Sleep* 9 (May 19, 2017): 151–61, http://doi.org/10.2147/NSS.S134864.

2. Lulu Xie et al., "Sleep Drives Metabolite Clearance from the Adult Brain," *Science* 342, no. 6156 (October 18, 2013): 373–77, http://doi .org/10.1126/science.1241224.

3. Zahid Saghir et al., "The Amygdala, Sleep Debt, Sleep Deprivation, and the Emotion of Anger: A Possible Connection," *Cureus* 10, no. 7 (July 2018): e2912, http://doi.org/10.7759/cureus.2912.

4. William D. S. Killgore, "Effects of Sleep Deprivation on Cognition," *Progress in Brain Research* 185 (2010): 105–29, http://doi.org/10.1016/ B978-0-444-53702-7.00007-5.

5. Hugh H. K. Fullagar et al., "Sleep and Athletic Performance: The Effects of Sleep Loss on Exercise Performance, and Physiological and Cognitive Responses to Exercise," *Sports Medicine* 45, no. 2 (February 2015): 161–86, http://doi.org/10.1007/s40279-014-0260-0.

6. Georges Copinschi, "Metabolic and Endocrine Effects of Sleep Deprivation," *Essential Psychopharmacology* 6, no. 6 (2005): 341–47, https://pubmed.ncbi .nlm.nih.gov/16459757/.

7. Michiaki Nagai, Satoshi Hoshide, and Kazuomi Kario, "Sleep Duration as a Risk Factor for Cardiovascular Disease—A Review of the Recent Literature," *Current Cardiology Reviews* 6, no. 1 (February 2010): 54–61, http://doi.org/10. 2174/157340310790231635.

8. Chun Seng Phua, Lata Jayaram, and Tissa Wijeratne, "Relationship between Sleep Duration and Risk Factors for Stroke," *Frontiers in Neurology* 8 (August 8, 2017): 392, http://doi.org/10.3389/fneur.2017.00392.

9. Erhard L. Haus and Michael H. Smolensky, "Shift Work and Cancer Risk: Potential Mechanistic Roles of Circadian Disruption, Light at Night, and Sleep Deprivation," *Sleep Medicine Reviews* 17, no. 4 (August 2013): 273–84, http://doi.org/10.1016/j.smrv.2012.08.003.

10. Yo-El S. Ju, Brendan P. Lucey, and David M. Holtzman, "Sleep and Alzheimer's Disease Pathology—A Bidirectional Relationship," *Nature Reviews Neurology* 10, no. 2 (February 2014): 115–19, http://doi.org/10.1038/ nrneurol.2013.269.

11. Matthew Walker, *Why We Sleep* (New York: Simon & Schuster, 2017), 158–60.

12. Serge M. Candeias and Udo Gaipl, "The Immune System in Cancer Prevention, Development and Therapy," *Anti-Cancer Agents in Medicinal Chemistry* 16, no. 1 (2016): 101–107, http://doi.org/10.2174/1871520615666150824153523.

13. Walker, *Why We Sleep*, 184–85.

14. Arisa Hirano et al., "DEC2 Modulates Orexin Expression and Regulates Sleep," *Proceedings of the National Academy of Sciences United States of America* 115, no. 13 (March 27, 2018): 3434–39, http://doi.org/10.1073/pnas.1801693115.

15. Walker, *Why We Sleep*, 146.

16. Emma Childs et al., "Association between ADORA2A and DRD2 Polymorphisms and Caffeine-Induced Anxiety," *Neuropsychopharmacology* 33, no. 12 (November 2008): 2791–800, http://doi.org/10.1038/npp.2008.17.

17. C. R. Jones et al., "Familial Advanced Sleep-Phase Syndrome: A Short-Period Circadian Rhythm Variant in Humans," *Nature Medicine* 5, no. 9 (September 1999): 1062–65, http://doi.org/10.1038/12502.

18. Zhi-Li Huang, Ze Zhang, and Wei-Min Qu, "Roles of Adenosine and Its Receptors in Sleep-Wake Regulation," *International Review of Neurobiology* 119 (2014): 349–71, http://doi.org/10.1016/B978-0-12-801022-8.00014-3.

19. Andrew J. K. Phillips et al., "Mammalian Sleep Dynamics: How Diverse Features Arise from a Common Physiological Framework," *PLOS Computational Biology* 6, no. 6 (June 24, 2010): e1000826, http://doi.org/10.1371/journal.pcbi.1000826.

20. Androniki Naska et al., "Siesta in Healthy Adults and Coronary Mortality in the General Population," *Archives of Internal Medicine* 167, no. 3 (February 12, 2007): 296–301, http://doi.org/10.1001/archinte.167.3.296.

CHAPTER 5

1. Ingrid H. Sarelius and U. Pohl, "Control of Muscle Blood Flow during Exercise: Local Factors and Integrative Mechanisms," *Acta Physiologica* 199, no. 4 (August 2010): 349–65, http://doi.org/10.1111/j.1748-1716.2010.02129.x.

CHAPTER 6

1. Liguo Sun et al., "Effects of Mechanical Stretch on Cell Proliferation and Matrix Formation of Mesenchymal Stem Cell and Anterior Cruciate Ligament Fibroblast," *Stem Cells International* (2016): 9842075, http://doi.org/10.1155/2016/9842075.

2. Kazuki Hotta et al., "Daily Muscle Stretching Enhances Blood Flow, Endothelial Function, Capillary, Vascular Volume and Connectivity in Aged Skeletal Muscle," *Journal of Physiology* 596, no. 10 (May 15, 2018): 1903–17, http://doi.org/10.1113/JP275459.

3. D. Knudson et al., "Acute Effects of Stretching Are Not Evident in the Kinematics of the Vertical Jump," *Journal of Strength and Conditioning Research* 15, no. 1 (February 2001): 98–101, https://pubmed.ncbi.nlm.nih.gov/11708715/.

4. P. J. McNair et al., "Stretching at the Ankle Joint: Viscoelastic Responses to Holds and Continuous Passive Motion," *Medicine and Science in Sport and Exercise* 33, no. 3 (March 2001): 354–58, http://doi .org/10.1097/00005768-200103000-00003.

5. Alexander M. Zollner et al., "Stretching Skeletal Muscle: Chronic Muscle Lengthening through Sarcomerogenesis," *PLOS ONE* 7, no. 10 (2012): e45661, http://doi.org/10.1371/journal.pone.0045661.

6. D. M. Medeiros and C. S. Lima, "Influence of Chronic Stretching on Muscle Performance: Systematic Review," *Human Movement Science* 54 (Aug. 2017): 220–29, http://doi.org/10.1016/j.humov.2017.05.006.

CHAPTER 10

1. Stoyan Dimitrov, Elaine Hulteng, and Suzi Hong, "Inflammation and Exercise: Inhibition of Monocytic Intracellular TNF Production by Acute Exercise Via B2-Adrenergic Activation," *Brain, Behavior, and Immunity* 61 (March 2017): 60–68, http://doi.org/10.1016/j.bbi.2016.12.017.

2. G. Howatson, D. Gaze, and K. A. van Someren, "The Efficacy of Ice Massage in the Treatment of Exercise-Induced Muscle Damage," *Scandinavian Journal of Medicine and Science in Sports* 15, no. 6 (December 2005): 416–22, http://doi.org/10.1111/j.1600-0838.2005.00437.x.

3. Ryo Takagi et al., "Influence of Icing on Muscle Regeneration after Crush Injury to Skeletal Muscles in Rats," *Journal of Applied Physiology* 110, no. 2 (February 2011): 382–88, http://doi.org/10.1152/japplphysiol.01187.2010.

4. Jan C. M. Prins et al., "Feasibility and Preliminary Effectiveness of Ice Therapy in Patients with an Acute Tear in the Gastrocnemius Muscle: A Pilot Randomized Controlled Trial," *Clinical Rehabilitation* 25, no. 5 (May 2011): 433–41, http://doi.org/10.1177/0269215510388312.

5. Ching-Yu Tseng et al., "Topical Cooling (Icing) Delays Recovery from Eccentric Exercise-Induced Muscle Damage," *Journal of Strength and Conditioning Research* 27, no. 5 (May 2013): 1354–61, http://doi.org/10.1519/JSC.0b013e318267a22c.

6. Naomi J. Crystal et al., "Effect of Cryotherapy on Muscle Recovery and Inflammation Following a Bout of Damaging Exercise," *European Journal of Applied Physiology* 113, no. 10 (October 2013): 2577–86, http://doi .org/10.1007/s00421-013-2693-9.

7. C. M. Bleakley et al., "Cryotherapy for Acute Ankle Sprains: A Randomised Controlled Study of Two Different Icing Protocols," *British Journal of Sports Medicine* 40, no. 8 (August 2006): 700–705, http://doi.org/10.1136/bjsm.2006.025932.

8. Ana Luiza Cabrera Martimbianco et al., "Effectiveness and Safety of Cryotherapy after Arthroscopic Anterior Cruciate Ligament Reconstruction: A Systematic Review of the Literature," *Physical Therapy in Sport* 15, no. 4 (November 2014): 261–68, http://doi.org/10.1016/j.ptsp.2014.02.008.

CHAPTER 17

1. Karen Briggs et al., "Prevalence of Acetabular Labral Tears in Asymptomatic Young Athletes," *British Journal of Sports Medicine* 51, no. 4 (2017): 303, http://doi.org/10.1136/bjsports-2016-097372.50.

2. A. J. J. Lee et al., "The Prevalence of Asymptomatic Labral Tears and Associated Pathology in a Young Asymptomatic Population," *Bone and Joint Journal* 97-B, no. 5 (May 2015): 623–27, http://doi.org/10.1302/0301-620X.97B5.35166.

3. Brad Register et al., "Prevalence of Abnormal Hip Findings in Asymptomatic Participants: A Prospective, Blinded Study," *American Journal of Sports Medicine* 40, no. 12 (December 2012): 2720–24, http://doi.org/10.1177/0363546512462124.

CHAPTER 18

1. Anny Sauvageau, Anne Desjarlais, and Stephanie Racette, "Deaths in a Head-Down Position: A Case Report and Review of the Literature," *Forensic Science, Medicine, and Pathology* 4, no. 1 (2008): 51–54, http://doi.org/10.1007/s12024-007-0031-4.

2. Julie M. Fritz et al., "Is There a Subgroup of Patients with Low Back Pain Likely to Benefit from Mechanical Traction? Results of a Randomized Clinical Trial and Subgrouping Analysis," *Spine* 32, no. 26 (December 15, 2007): E793–E800, http://doi.org/10.1097/BRS.0b013e31815d001a.

3. Andrew J. Schoenfeld and Bradley K. Weiner, "Treatment of Lumbar Disc Herniation: Evidenced-Based Practice," *International Journal of General Medicine* 3 (July 21, 2010): 209–14, http://doi.org/10.2147/ijgm.s12270.

CHAPTER 19

1. William R. Vanwye, Alyssa M. Weatherholt, and Alan E. Mikesky, "Blood Flow Restriction Training: Implementation into Clinical Practice," *International Journal of Exercise Science* 10, no. 5 (September 1, 2017): 649–54, https://www.ncbi.nlm.nih.gov/pmc/articles/PMC5609669/.

CHAPTER 20

1. C. K. Wong et al., "Natural History of Frozen Shoulder: Fact or Fiction? A Systematic Review," *Physiotherapy* 103, no. 1 (March 2017): 40–47, http://doi.org/10.1016/j.physio.2016.05.009.

APPENDIX I

1. Brad J. Schoenfeld, "Squatting Kinematics and Kinetics and Their Application to Exercise Performance," *Journal of Strength and Conditioning Research* 24, no. 12 (December 2010): 3497–506, http://doi.org/10.1519/JSC.0b013e3181bac2d7.

BIBLIOGRAPHY

Al-Aama, Tareef. "Falls in the Elderly: Spectrum and Prevention." *Canadian Family Physician* 57, no. 7 (July 2011): 771–76. https://pubmed.ncbi.nlm.nih.gov/21753098/

American Cancer Society. "Recombinant Bovine Growth Hormone." Last modified September 10, 2014. https://www.cancer.org/cancer/cancer-causes/recombinant-bovine-growth-hormone.html

Amin, Moamen, Suganthiny Jeyaganth, and Armen Aprikian. "Dietary Habits and Prostate Cancer Detection: A Case-Control Study." *Canadian Urological Association Journal* 2, no. 5 (October 2008): 510–15. https://www.ncbi.nlm.nih.gov/pmc/articles/PMC2572247/#__ffn_sectitle

Andrich, David E., Marie-Eve Filion, Margo Woods, Johanna T. Dwyer, Sherwood L. Gorbach, Barry R. Goldin, Herman Adlercreutz, and Mylene Aubertin-Leheudre. "Relationship between Essential Amino Acids and Muscle Mass, Independent of Habitual Diets, in Pre- and Post-Menopausal US Women." *International Journal of Food Sciences and Nutrition* 62, no. 7 (November 2011): 719–24. https://doi.org/10.3109/09637486.2011.573772

Basu, Sanjay, Paula Yoffee, Nancy Hills, and Robert H. Lustig. "The Relationship of Sugar to Population-Level Diabetes Prevalence: An Econometric Analysis of Repeated Cross-Sectional Data." *PLOS ONE* 8, no. 2 (February 27, 2013): e57873. https://doi.org/10.1371/journal.pone.0057873

Bennett, Mary Payne, and Cecile Lengacher. "Humor and Laughter May Influence Health: III. Laughter and Health Outcomes." *Evidence-Based Complementary and Alternative Medicine* 5, no. 1 (March 2008): 37–40. https://doi.org/10.1093/ecam/nem041

Bleakley, C. M., S. M. McDonough, D. C. MacAuley, and J. Bjordal. "Cryotherapy for Acute Ankle Sprains: A Randomised Controlled Study of Two Different Icing Protocols." *British Journal of Sports Medicine* 40, no. 8 (August 2006): 700–705. http://dx.doi.org/10.1136/bjsm.2006.025932

Bouvard, Veronique, Dana Loomis, Kathryn Z. Guyton, Yann Grosse, Fatiha El Ghissassi, Lamia Bengrahim-Tallaa, Neela Guha, Heidi Mattock, and Kurt Straif. "Carcinogenicity of Consumption of Red and Processed Meat." *Lancet Oncology* 16, no. 16 (December 2015): 1599–600. https://doi.org/10.1016/s1470-2045(15)00444-1

Brasky, Theodore M., Emily White, and Chi-Ling Chen. "Long-Term, Supplemental, One-Carbon Metabolism-Related Vitamin B Use in Relation to Lung Cancer Risk in the Vitamins and Lifestyle (VITAL) Cohort." *Journal of Clinical Oncology* 35, no. 30 (October 20, 2017): 3440–48. https://ascopubs.org/doi/10.1200/JCO.2017.72.7735

Briggs, Karen, Marc Philippon, Charles Ho, and Shannen McNamara. "Prevalence of Acetabular Labral Tears in Asymptomatic Young Athletes." *British Journal of Sports Medicine* 51, no. 4 (2017): 303. http://dx.doi.org/10.1136/bjsports-2016-097372.50

Bureau of Labor Statistics. "2016 Survey of Occupational Injuries and Illnesses Charts Package." November 9, 2017. https://www.bls.gov/iif/osch0060.pdf

Candeias, Serge M., and Udo Gaipl. "The Immune System in Cancer Prevention, Development and Therapy." *Anti-Cancer Agents in Medicinal Chemistry* 16, no. 1 (2016): 101–107. http://doi.org/10.2174/1871520615666150824153523

Capstone Partners, Investment Banking Advisers. "Outpatient Physical Therapy, Q1 2017." https://capstoneheadwaters.com/sites/default/files/Capstone%20Outpatient%20Physical%20Therapy%20M&A%20Report_1Q%202017_0.pdf

Chen, Mu, Yanping Li, Qi Sun, An Pan, JoAnn E. Manson, Kathryn M. Rexrode, Walter C. Willett, Eric B. Rimm, and Frank B. Hu. "Dairy Fat and Risk of Cardiovascular Disease in 3 Cohorts of US Adults." *American Journal of Clinical Nutrition* 104, no. 5 (November 2016): 1209–17. http://doi.org/10.3945/ajcn.116.134460

Childs, Emma, Christa Hohoff, Jurgen Deckert, Ke Xu, Judith Badner, and Harriet de Wit. "Association between ADORA2A and DRD2 Polymorphisms and Caffeine-Induced Anxiety." *Neuropsychopharmacology* 33, no. 12 (November 2008): 2791–800. http://doi.org/10.1038/npp.2008.17

Copinschi, Georges. "Metabolic and Endocrine Effects of Sleep Deprivation." *Essential Psychopharmacology* 6, no. 6 (2005): 341–47. https://pubmed.ncbi.nlm.nih.gov/16459757/

Costa e Silva, Lara, Maria Isabel Fragoso, and Julia Teles. "Physical Activity-Related Injury Profile in Children and Adolescents according to Their Age, Maturation, and Level of Sports Participation." *Sports Health* 9, no. 2 (March–April 2017): 118–25. http://doi.org/10.1177/1941738116686964

Crystal, Naomi J., David H. Townson, Summer B. Cook, and Dain P. La-Roche. "Effect of Cryotherapy on Muscle Recovery and Inflammation Following a Bout of Damaging Exercise." *European Journal of Applied Physiology* 113, no. 10 (October 2013): 2577–86. http://doi.org/10.1007/s00421-013-2693-9

Delimaris, Ioannis. "Adverse Effects Associated with Protein Intake above the Recommended Dietary Allowance for Adults." *ISRN Nutrition* (July 18, 2013): 126929. http://doi.org/10.5402/2013/126929

Delitto, Anthony, Sara R. Piva, Charity G. Moore, Julie M. Fritz, Stephen R. Wisniewski, Deborah A. Josbeno, Mark Fye, and William C. Welch. "Surgery versus Nonsurgical Treatment of Lumbar Spinal Stenosis: A Randomized Trial." *Annals of Internal Medicine* 162, no. 7 (April 7, 2015): 465–73. http://doi.org/10.7326/M14-1420

Dimitrov, Stoyan, Elaine Hulteng, and Suzi Hong. "Inflammation and Exercise: Inhibition of Monocytic Intracellular TNF Production by Acute Exercise Via B2-Adrenergic Activation." *Brain, Behavior, and Immunity* 61 (March 2017): 60–68. http://doi.org/10.1016/j.bbi.2016.12.017

Erickson, Kirk I., Regina L. Leckie, and Andrea M. Weinstein. "Physical Activity, Fitness, and Gray Matter Volume." *Neurobiology of Aging* 35, no. 2 (September 2014): S20–S28. http://doi.org/10.1016/j.neurobiolaging.2014.03.034

Erickson, Kirk I., Michelle W. Voss, Ruchika Shaurya Prakash, Chandramallika Basak, Amanda Szabo, Laura Chaddock, Jennifer S. Kim, et al. "Exercise Training Increases Size of Hippocampus and Improves Memory." *Proceedings of the National Academy of Sciences of the United States of America* 108, no. 7 (February 15, 2011): 3017–22. http://doi.org/10.1073/pnas.1015950108

Esselstyn, Caldwell B. Jr., Gina Gendy, Jonathan Doyle, Mladen Golubic, and Michael F. Roizen. "A Way to Reverse CAD?" *Journal of Family Practice* 63, no. 7 (July 2014): 356–64b. https://pubmed.ncbi.nlm.nih.gov/25198208/

Feskanich, Diane, Walter C. Willett, Meir J. Stampfer, and Graham A. Colditz. "Milk, Dietary Calcium, and Bone Fractures in Women: A 12-Year Prospective Study." *American Journal of Public Health* 87, no. 6 (June 1997): 992–97. http://doi.org/10.2105/aiph.87.6.992

Fritz, Julie M., Gerard P. Brennan, and Stephen J. Hunter. "Physical Therapy or Advanced Imaging as First Management Strategy Following a New Consultation for Low Back Pain in Primary Care: Associations with Future Health Care Utilization and Charges." *Health Services Research* 50, no. 6 (March 16, 2015): 1927–40. http://doi.org/10.1111/1475-6773.12301

Fritz, Julie M., Weston Lindsay, James W. Matheson, Gerard P. Brennan, Stephen J. Hunter, Steve D. Moffit, Aaron Swalberg, and Brian Rodriquez. "Is

There a Subgroup of Patients with Low Back Pain Likely to Benefit from Mechanical Traction? Results of a Randomized Clinical Trial and Subgrouping Analysis." *Spine* 32, no. 26 (December 15, 2007): E793–E800. http://doi.org/10.1097/BRS.0b013e31815d001a

Fullagar, Hugh H. K., Sabrina Skorski, Rob Duffield, Daniel Hammes, Aaron J. Coutts, and Tim Meyer. "Sleep and Athletic Performance: The Effects of Sleep Loss on Exercise Performance, and Physiological and Cognitive Responses to Exercise." *Sports Medicine* 45, no. 2 (February 2015): 161–86. http://doi.org/10.1007/s40279-014-0260-0

Gao, Xiang, Michael P. LaValley, and Katherine L. Tucker. "Prospective Studies of Dairy Product and Calcium Intakes and Prostate Cancer Risk: A Meta-Analysis." *Journal of the National Cancer Institute* 97, no. 23 (December 7, 2005): 1768–77. http://doi.org/10.1093/jnci/dji402

Haus, Erhard L., and Michael H. Smolensky. "Shift Work and Cancer Risk: Potential Mechanistic Roles of Circadian Disruption, Light at Night, and Sleep Deprivation." *Sleep Medicine Reviews* 17, no. 4 (August 2013): 273–84. http://doi.org/10.1016/j.smrv.2012.08.003

Hirano, Arisa, Pei-Ken Hsu, Luoying Zhang, Lijuan Xing, Thomas McMahon, Maya Yamazaki, Louis P. Ptacek, and Ying-Hui Fu. "DEC2 Modulates Orexin Expression and Regulates Sleep." *Proceedings of the National Academy of Sciences United States of America* 115, no. 13 (March 27, 2018): 3434–39. http://doi.org/10.1073/pnas.1801693115

Hotta, Kazuki, Bradley J. Behnke, Bahram Arjmandi, Payal Ghosh, Bei Chen, Rachael Brooks, Joshua J. Maraj et al. "Daily Muscle Stretching Enhances Blood Flow, Endothelial Function, Capillary, Vascular Volume and Connectivity in Aged Skeletal Muscle." *Journal of Physiology* 596, no. 10 (May 15, 2018): 1903–17. http://doi.org/10.1113/JP275459

Howatson, G., D. Gaze, and K. A. van Someren. "The Efficacy of Ice Massage in the Treatment of Exercise-Induced Muscle Damage." *Scandinavian Journal of Medicine and Science in Sports* 15, no. 6 (Dec. 2005): 416–22. http://doi.org/10.1111/j.1600-0838.2005.00437.x

Hu, Frank B. "Plant-Based Foods and Prevention of Cardiovascular Disease: An Overview." *American Journal of Clinical Nutrition* 78, no. 3 (suppl) (September 2003): 544S–51S. http://doi.org/10.1093/ajcn/78.3.544S

Huang, Zhi-Li, Ze Zhang, and Wei-Min Qu. "Roles of Adenosine and Its Receptors in Sleep-Wake Regulation." *International Review of Neurobiology* 119 (2014): 349–71. http://doi.org/10.1016/B978-0-12-801022-8.00014-3

Jenkins, David J., Cyril W. Kendall, D. G. Popovich, E. Vidhen, C. C. Mehling, Vladimir Vuksan, and T. P. Ransom. "Effect of a Very-High-Fiber Vegetable, Fruit, and Nut Diet on Serum Lipids and Colonic Function." *Metabolism* 50, no. 4 (April 2001): 494–503. http://doi.org/10.1053/meta.2001.21037

Jiang, Yan, Yong Pan, Patrea R. Rhea, Lin Tan, Mihai Gagea, Lorenzo Cohen, Susan M. Fischer, and Peiying Yang. "A Sucrose-Enriched Diet Promotes Tumorigenesis in Mammary Gland in Part through the 12-Lipoxygenase Pathway." *Cancer Research* 76, no. 1 (January 1, 2016): 24–29. http://doi .org/10.1158/0008-5472.CAN-14-3432

Jones, C. R., S. S. Campbell, S. E. Zone, F. Cooper, A. DeSano, P. J. Murphy, B. Jones, L. Czajkowski, and L. J. Ptacek. "Familial Advanced Sleep-Phase Syndrome: A Short-Period Circadian Rhythm Variant in Humans." *Nature Medicine* 5, no. 9 (September 1999): 1062–65. http://doi.org/10.1038/12502

Ju, Yo-El S., Brendan P. Lucey, and David M. Holtzman. "Sleep and Alzheimer's Disease Pathology—A Bidirectional Relationship." *Nature Reviews Neurology* 10, no. 2 (February 2014): 115–19. http://doi.org/10.1038/nrneurol.2013.269

Kamangar, Farin, and Ashkan Emadi. "Vitamin and Mineral Supplements: Do We Really Need Them?" *International Journal of Preventive Medicine* 3, no. 3 (March 2012): 221–26. https://pubmed.ncbi.nlm.nih.gov/22448315/

Killgore, William D. S. "Effects of Sleep Deprivation on Cognition." *Progress in Brain Research* 185 (2010): 105–29. http://doi.org/10.1016/B978-0-444-53702-7.00007-5

Knudson, D., K. Bennett, R. Corn, D. Leick, and C. Smith. "Acute Effects of Stretching Are Not Evident in the Kinematics of the Vertical Jump." *Journal of Strength and Conditioning Research* 15, no. 1 (February 2001): 98–101. https://pubmed.ncbi.nlm.nih.gov/11708715/

Kramer, Arthur F., Kirk I. Erickson, and Stanley J. Colcombe. "Exercise, Cognition, and the Aging Brain." *Journal of Applied Physiology* 101, no. 4 (October 2006): 1237–42. http://doi.org/10.1152/japplphysiol.00500.2006

Lanou, Amy Joy. "Should Dairy Be Recommended as Part of a Healthy Vegetarian Diet? Counterpoint." *American Journal of Clinical Nutrition* 89, no. 5 (May 2009): 1638S–42S. http://doi.org/10.3945/ajcn.2009.26736P

Lanou, Amy Joy, Susan E. Berkow, and Neal D. Barnard. "Calcium, Dairy Products, and Bone Health in Children and Young Adults: A Reevaluation of the Evidence." *Pediatrics* 115, no. 3 (March 2005): 736–43. http://doi .org/10.1542/peds.2004-0548

Larsson, Susanna C., Leif Bergkvist, and Alicja Wolk. "Milk and Lactose Intakes and Ovarian Cancer Risk in the Swedish Mammography Cohort." *American Journal of Clinical Nutrition* 80, no. 5 (November 2004): 1353–57. http://doi .org/10.1093/ajcn/80.5.1353

Lee, A. J. J., P. Armour, D. Thind, M. H. Coates, and A. C. L. Kang. "The Prevalence of Asymptomatic Labral Tears and Associated Pathology in a Young Asymptomatic Population." *Bone and Joint Journal* 97-B, no. 5 (May 2015): 623–27. http://doi.org/10.1302/0301-620X.97B5.35166

Lustig, Robert H. "Childhood Obesity: Behavioral Aberration or Biochemical Drive? Reinterpreting the First Law of Thermodynamics." *Nature Clinical Practice Endocrinology and Metabolism* 2, no. 8 (August 2006): 447–58. http://doi.org/10.1038/ncpendmet0220

Martimbianco, Ana Luiza Cabrera, Brenda Nazare Gomes da Silva, Alan Pedrosa, Viegas de Carvalho, Valter Silva, Maria Regina Torloni, and Maria Stella Peccin. "Effectiveness and Safety of Cryotherapy after Arthroscopic Anterior Cruciate Ligament Reconstruction. A Systematic Review of the Literature." *Physical Therapy in Sport* 15, no. 4 (November 2014): 261–68. http://doi.org/10.1016/j.ptsp.2014.02.008

McCann, Susan E., Justine Hays, Charlotte W. Baumgart, Edward H. Weiss, Song Yao, and Christine B. Ambrosone. "Usual Consumption of Specific Dairy Foods Is Associated with Breast Cancer in the Roswell Park Cancer Institute Databank and BioRepository." *Current Developments in Nutrition* 1, no. 3 (February 16, 2017): e000422. http://doi.org/10.3945/cdn.117.000422

McNair, P. J., E. W. Dombroski, D. J. Hewson, and S. N. Stanley. "Stretching at the Ankle Joint: Viscoelastic Responses to Holds and Continuous Passive Motion." *Medicine and Science in Sport and Exercise* 33, no. 3 (March 2001): 354–58. http://doi.org/10.1097/00005768-200103000-00003

Medeiros, D. M., and C. S. Lima. "Influence of Chronic Stretching on Muscle Performance: Systematic Review." *Human Movement Science* 54 (August 2017): 220–29. http://doi.org/10.1016/j.humov.2017.05.006

Medic, Goran, Micheline Wille, and Michiel E. H. Hemels. "Short- and Long-Term Health Consequences of Sleep Disruption." *Nature and Science of Sleep* 9 (May 19, 2017): 151–61. http://doi.org/10.2147/NSS.S134864

MedRisk 2018 Industry Trends Report, Physical Medicine and Workers' Comp. "Workers' Comp Costs: Why Physical Therapy Is Bigger Than You Think (Part 1 of 2)." https://www.medrisknet.com/workers-comp-costs-why-physical-therapy-is-bigger-than-you-think-part-1-of-2/

Moss, Michael. *Salt, Sugar, Fat: How the Food Giants Hooked Us.* New York: Random House, 2013.

Nagai, Michiaki, Satoshi Hoshide, and Kazuomi Kario. "Sleep Duration as a Risk Factor for Cardiovascular Disease—A Review of the Recent Literature." *Current Cardiology Reviews* 6, no. 1 (February 2010): 54–61. http://doi.org/10.2174/157340310790231635

Naska, Androniki, Eleni Oikonomou, Antonia Trichopoulou, Theodora Psalto-poulou, and Dimitrios Trichopoulos. "Siesta in Healthy Adults and Coronary Mortality in the General Population." *Archives of Internal Medicine* 167, no. 3 (February 12, 2007): 296–301. http://doi.org/10.1001/archinte.167.3.296

Nasser, Munir J. "How to Approach the Problem of Low Back Pain: An Over-view." *Journal of Family and Community Medicine* 12, no. 1 (January–April 2005): 3–9. https://www.ncbi.nlm.nih.gov/pmc/articles/PMC3410134/?report=classic

Nestle, Marion. "Food Lobbies, the Food Pyramid, and U.S. Nutrition Policy." *International Journal of Health Services* 23, no. 3 (July 1, 1993): 483–96. http://doi.org/10.2190/32F2-2PFB-MEG7-8HPU

Phillips, Andrew J. K., Peter A. Robinson, David J. Kedziora, and Romesh G. Abeysuriya. "Mammalian Sleep Dynamics: How Diverse Features Arise from a Common Physiological Framework." *PLOS Computational Biology* 6, no. 6 (June 24, 2010): e1000826. http://doi.org/10.1371/journal.pcbi.1000826

Phua, Chun Seng, Lata Jayaram, and Tissa Wijeratne. "Relationship between Sleep Duration and Risk Factors for Stroke." *Frontiers in Neurology* 8 (August 8, 2017): 392. http://doi.org/10.3389/fneur.2017.00392

Prins, Jan C. M., Janine H. Stubbe, Nico L. U. van Meeteren, Frans A. Schef-fers, and Martien C. J. M. van Dongen. "Feasibility and Preliminary Effec-tiveness of Ice Therapy in Patients with an Acute Tear in the Gastrocnemius Muscle: A Pilot Randomized Controlled Trial." *Clinical Rehabilitation* 25, no. 5 (May 2011): 433–41. http://doi.org/10.1177/0269215510388312

Rao, Nisha, Henry A. Spiller, Nichole L. Hodges, Thiphalak Chounthirath, Marcel J. Casavant, Amrit K. Kamboj, and Gary A. Smith. "An Increase in Dietary Supplement Exposures Reported to US Poison Control Centers." *Journal of Medical Toxicology* 13, no. 3 (September 2017): 227–37. http://doi.org/10.1007/s13181-017-0623-7

Register, Brad, Andrew T. Pennock, Charles P. Ho, Colin D. Strickland, Ashur Lawand, and Marc J. Philippon. "Prevalence of Abnormal Hip Find-ings in Asymptomatic Participants: A Prospective, Blinded Study." *American Journal of Sports Medicine* 40, no. 12 (December 2012): 2720–24. http://doi.org/10.1177/0363546512462124

Saghir, Zahid, Javeria N. Syeda, Adnan S. Muhammad, and Tareg H. Balla. "The Amygdala, Sleep Debt, Sleep Deprivation, and the Emotion of Anger: A Possible Connection." *Cureus* 10, no. 7 (July 2018): e2912. http://doi.org/10.7759/cureus.2912

Sarelius, Ingrid H., and U. Pohl. "Control of Muscle Blood Flow during Ex-ercise: Local Factors and Integrative Mechanisms." *Acta Physiologica* 199, no. 4 (August 2010): 349–65. http://doi.org/10.1111/j.1748-1716.2010.02129.x

Sauvageau, Anny, Anne Desjarlais, and Stephanie Racette. "Deaths in a Head-Down Position: A Case Report and Review of the Literature." *Forensic Science, Medicine, and Pathology* 4, no. 1 (2008): 51–54. http://doi.org/10.1007/s12024-007-0031-4

Sawyer, Bradley, and McDermott, Daniel. "How Does the Quality of the U.S. Healthcare System Compare to Other Countries?" *Peterson-KFF Health System Tracker*, March 28, 2019. https://www.healthsystemstracker.org/chart-collection/quality-u-s-healthcare-system-compare-countries/#item-start

Schoenfeld, Andrew J., and Bradley K. Weiner. "Treatment of Lumbar Disc Herniation: Evidenced-Based Practice." *International Journal of General Medicine* 3 (July 21, 2010): 209–14. http://doi.org/10.2147/ijgm.s12270

Schoenfeld, Brad J. "Squatting Kinematics and Kinetics and Their Application to Exercise Performance." *Journal of Strength and Conditioning Research* 24, no. 12 (December 2010): 3497–506. http://doi.org/10.1519/JSC.0b013e3181bac2d7

Sellmeyer, Deborah E., Katie L. Stone, A. Sebastian, and Steven R. Cummings. "A High Ratio of Dietary Animal to Vegetable Protein Increases the Rate of Bone Loss and the Risk of Fracture in Postmenopausal Women." *American Journal of Clinical Nutrition* 73, no. 1 (January 2001): 118–22. http://doi.org/10.1093/ajcn/73.1.118

Sheu, Yahtyng, Li-Hui Chen, and Holly Hedegaard. "Sports- and Recreation-Related Injury Episodes in the United States, 2011–2014." *National Health Statistics Reports* 99 (Nov. 18, 2016): 1–12. https://pubmed.ncbi.nlm.nih.gov/27906643/

Song, Yan, Jorge E. Chavarro, Yin Cao, Weiliang Qiu, Lorelei Mucci, Howard D. Sesso, Meir J. Stampfer, et al. "Whole Milk Intake Is Associated with Prostate Cancer–Specific Mortality among U.S. Male Physicians." *Journal of Nutrition* 143, no. 2 (February 2013): 189–96. http://doi.org/10.3945/jn.112.168484

Stang, Andreas, Wolfgang Ahrens, Cornelia Baumgardt-Elms, Christa Stegmaier, Hiltrud Merzenich, Michael de Vrese, Jurgen Schrezenmeir, and Karl-Heinz Jockel. "Adolescent Milk Fat and Galactose Consumption and Testicular Germ Cell Cancer." *Cancer Epidemiology, Biomarkers & Prevention* 15, no. 11 (November 2006): 2189–95. http://doi.org/10.1158/1055-9965.EPI-06-0372

Stern, Aaron. "Food Industry Influence on Dietary Advice in the United States." *Proceedings of the National Conference on Undergraduate Research*, April 7–9, 2016, University of North Carolina Asheville. https://www.ncurproceedings.org/ojs/index.php/NCUR2016/article/view/1706/903

Sun, Liguo, Ling Qu, Rui Zhu, Hongguo Li, Yingsen Xue, Xincheng Liu, Jiabing Fan, and Hongbin Fan. "Effects of Mechanical Stretch on Cell Proliferation and Matrix Formation of Mesenchymal Stem Cell and Anterior Cruciate Ligament Fibroblast." *Stem Cells International* (2016): 9842075. http://doi.org/10.1155/2016/9842075

Swan, Shanna, Fei Liu, James W. Overstreet, C. Brazil, and Niels Erik Skakkebaek. "Growth Hormones Fed to Beef Cattle Damage Human Health." *Organic Consumers Association*, May 1, 2007. https://www.organicconsumers.org/scientific/growth-hormones-fed-beef-cattle-damage-human-health

Swan, Shanna, Fei Liu, James W. Overstreet, C. Brazil, and Niels Erik Skakkebaek. "Semen Quality of Fertile US Males in Relation to Their Mother's Beef Consumption during Pregnancy." *Human Reproduction* 22, no. 6 (June 2007): 1497–502. http://doi.org/10.1093/humrep/dem068

Takagi, Ryo, Naoto Fujita, Takamitsu Arakawa, Shigeo Kawada, Naokata Ishii, and Akinori Miki. "Influence of Icing on Muscle Regeneration after Crush Injury to Skeletal Muscles in Rats." *Journal of Applied Physiology* 110, no. 2 (February 2011): 382–88. http://doi.org/10.1152/japplphysiol.01187.2010

Tanne, Janice. "US Gets Mediocre Results Despite High Spending on Health Care." *British Medical Journal* 333, no. 7570 (September 30, 2006): 672. https://www.ncbi.nlm.nih.gov/pmc/articles/PMC1584360/

Tseng, Ching-Yu, Jo-Ping Lee, Yung-Shen Tsai, Shin-Da Lee, Chung-Lan Kao, Te-Chih Liu, Cheng-Hsiu Lai, M. Brennan Harris, and Chia-Hua Kuo. "Topical Cooling (Icing) Delays Recovery from Eccentric Exercise-Induced Muscle Damage." *Journal of Strength and Conditioning Research* 27, no. 5 (May 2013): 1354–61. http://doi.org/10.1519/JSC.0b013e318267a22c

Vanwye, William R., Alyssa M. Weatherholt, and Alan E. Mikesky. "Blood Flow Restriction Training: Implementation into Clinical Practice." *International Journal of Exercise Science* 10, no. 5 (September 1, 2017): 649–54. https://www.ncbi.nlm.nih.gov/pmc/articles/PMC5609669/

Volkow, Nora D., Gene-Jack Wang, Joanna S. Fowler, Dardo Tomasi, and Ruben Baler. "Food and Drug Reward: Overlapping Circuits in Human Obesity and Addiction." *Current Topics in Behavioral Neurosciences* 11 (2012): 1–24. http://doi.org/10.1007/7854_2011_169

Walker, Matthew. *Why We Sleep.* New York: Simon & Schuster, 2017.

Wang, Zeneng, Nathalie Bergeron, Bruce S. Levison, Xinmin S. Li, Sally Chiu, Xun Jia, Robert A. Koeth, et al. "Impact of Chronic Dietary Red Meat, White Meat, or Non-Meat Protein on Trimethylamine N-Oxide Metabolism and Renal Excretion in Healthy Men and Women." *European Heart Journal* 40, no. 7 (February 14, 2019): 583–94. http://doi.org/10.1093/eurheartj/ehy799

Wong, C. K., W. N. Levine, K. Deo, R. S. Kesting, E. A. Mercer, G. A. Schram, and B. L. Strang. "Natural History of Frozen Shoulder: Fact or Fiction? A Systematic Review." *Physiotherapy* 103, no. 1 (March 2017): 40–47. http://doi.org/10.1016/j.physio.2016.05.009

Xie, Lulu, Hongyi Kang, Qiwu Xu, Michael J. Chen, Yonghong Liao, Meenakshisundaram Thiyagarajan, John O'Donnell, et al. "Sleep Drives Metabolite Clearance from the Adult Brain." *Science* 342, no. 6156 (October 18, 2013): 373–77. http://doi.org/10.1126/science.1241224

Yang, Quanhe, Zefeng Zhang, Edward W. Gregg, W. Dana Flanders, Robert Merritt, and Frank B. Hu. "Added Sugar Intake and Cardiovascular Diseases Mortality among US Adults." *JAMA Internal Medicine* 174, no. 4 (April 2014): 516–24. http://doi.org/10.1001/jamainternmed.2013.13563

Zollner, Alexander M., Oscar J. Abilez, Markus Bol, and Ellen Kuhl. "Stretching Skeletal Muscle: Chronic Muscle Lengthening through Sarcomerogenesis." *PLOS ONE* 7, no. 10 (2012): e45661. http://doi.org/10.1371/journal.pone.0045661

INDEX

ABOUT THE AUTHOR

Mark Salamon is a physical therapist with twenty-five years of experience teaching young athletes, middle-aged weekend warriors, workers injured on the job, and senior citizens how to restore their lives after injuries or surgeries. He earned a bachelor's in mechanical engineering from the University of Maryland in 1987, and a master's in physical therapy from Temple University in 1995. He honed his sense of humor by raising three daughters with his wife, Melissa, and has published more than sixty humorous articles in publications such as *The Haven* and *The Scene and Heard*. He was named a top writer in satire on Medium, and has helped more than twenty thousand patients decrease their anxiety and frustration by making them laugh.